The VBAC Companion

OTHER BOOKS BY DIANA KORTE

Every Woman's Body

A Good Birth, A Safe Birth
CO-AUTHORED BY
ROBERTA M. SCAER

The VBAC Companion

The Expectant Mother's Guide to Vaginal Birth After Cesarean

Diana Korte

The Harvard Common Press

Boston, Massachusetts

618.4
Kor

The author of this book is not a physician. All matters regarding your health require medical supervision. The suggestions contained in this book are not substitutes for professional medical advice. You should consult your physician before you follow suggestions in this book. The author and publishers disclaim any liability arising, whether directly or indirectly, from the use of this book.

The Harvard Common Press
535 Albany Street
Boston, Massachusetts 02118

Copyright © 1997 by The Harvard Common Press

Illustrations copyright © 1997 by Kathleen Gray Farthing

Printed in the United States of America
Printed on acid-free paper

Library of Congress Cataloging-in-Publication Data
Korte, Diana.
  The VBAC companion : the expectant mother's guide to vaginal birth after cesarean / Diana Korte.
      p. cm.
  Includes bibliographical references and index.
  ISBN 1-55832-128-4 (hbk. : alk. paper). — ISBN 1-55832-129-2 (pbk. : alk. paper)
  I. Title.
RG761.K67   1997
618'.4—dc21   97-31338
                                                                CIP

Special bulk-order discounts are available on this and other Harvard Common Press books. Companies and organizations may purchase books for premiums or for resale, or may arrange a custom edition, by contacting the Marketing Director at the address above.

Cover design and text design by Joyce C. Weston
Illustrations by Kathleen Gray Farthing

10 9 8 7 6 5 4 3 2 1

To my very sweet S, I did it all for you.

*To all the women who ever dreamed of having a
VBAC the next time, and to the VBAC pioneers who
cleared the path for everyone else.*

Contents

Acknowledgments

I would like to acknowledge the enormous help given to me in creating this book. First, my heartfelt thanks to my family: my husband, children, children-in-law, and grandchildren. They all have educated me by their very presence about the value of the process of birth and how it affects the kind of people we become.

Special mention and wild appreciation goes to publisher Bruce Shaw and his outstanding staff at the Harvard Common Press, including Dan, Chris, Holly, and Laura, for their enthusiasm, good will, and efficiency. (It's not always easy for a book publishing company to provide all three.) Much praise also to editor Leslie Baker for her clear thinking and to book doctor Nellie Sabin for keeping me fair.

Grateful appreciation goes to Kathleen Gray Farthing, who helped me more than any other person with her knowledge of VBACs. We can all thank her for the beautiful illustrations in this book as well. Gratitude also to Valerie El Halta for her "posterior" information.

Boulder pathologist John Meyer came through again by reviewing the book's illustrations. Words of wisdom from Nancy Wainer Cohen were invaluable, and Ruth Ancheta, Bruce Flamm, Roberta Gehrke, Nicette Jukelevics, and Jan Tritten each alerted me to something I might otherwise have overlooked. I thank them all.

As always, I am grateful for an international network of researchers. Much of the book is based on hundreds of medical journal articles, many of which are listed in the Bibliographic References. My thanks, too, to the healthcare statisticians in other countries who provided information about VBACs and childbirth practices. A special thank you goes to Norway. Under the guidance of Ole-Henrik Edland of the Medical Birth Registry of Norway, the Norwegians compiled their VBAC statistics for the first time.

Much of the information that includes national healthcare percentages came from the U.S. government, often from the National Center for Health Statistics (NCHS). I am particularly indebted to NCHS's Sally Clarke Curtin, Paul Placek, and Sam Notzon. Among the other people and organizations to whom I say thanks for information are Kimberly Patamia at the American College of Nurse-Midwives and Greg Phillips and Barbara Awaakye at the American College of Obstetricians and Gynecologists.

The more than one hundred VBAC letters I received were solicited using a variety of resources, including the Internet, a number of different publications, and fliers that I sent hither and yon. I thank everyone at the Internet sites that mentioned my quest for VBAC stories: Amazon.com, Family.com, OBCNews@efn.org (Donna Dolezal Zelzer), and ParentsPlace.com (Jackie Needleman), as well as any other web sites that posted my request. I'm also grateful to all the publications and organizations that put the word out for me, including *The Clarion,* a quarterly newsletter published by ICAN (the International Cesarean Awareness Network); *The Compleat Mother;* the *Los Angeles Times* Syndicate; *Michigan Friends of Midwives Newsletter;* the *Midwifery Task Force Newsletter; NAPSAC News,* published by the International Association of Parents and Professionals for Safe Alternatives in Childbirth; *Northwest Baby & Child;* and *Special Delivery,* the magazine published by the Association of Labor Assistants and Childbirth Educators (ALACE). Speaking of publications, a special thank you to Peggy O'Mara at *Mothering* magazine for publishing my original VBAC article, which—as it turned out—was the beginning of this book.

Appreciation goes to the following individuals and organizations who distributed my fliers and were helpful in other ways, too: Emily Aldrich; Australia's BACUP (Birth After Cesarean Unlimited Possibilities) and Anne Notarpietro; Birth Works; Canada's Susan Martensen and the Association of Ontario Midwives in Toronto; Martha Del Giudice; Pam Eades; England's Alliance for the Improvement of Maternity Services, M.C. Bradshaw, Caroline Flint,

Marjorie Tew, and VBAC Information and Support; Catherine Fuhrmann; Diane Goslin; La Leche League's Mary Ann Kerwin, Kathy Lange, and Katrina Switzer; Yvonne Cryns of the Midwives Alliance of North America (MANA); Willi Nolan at Biobiz; Jennifer Nunn and Doulas of North America; Debra O'Conner; Alison Osborne; Carole Summer; and Sunday Tortelli. My apologies and belated thanks to anyone I've unintentionally overlooked.

And, finally, I say thank you to all the women who sent me their stories—whether they had VBACs or not—and who contributed to the "heart" of the book. They are listed alphabetically.

Wendy Allen
Patience Anders
Cynthia Van Duyne Arthur
Jodi Barnett
Patricia-Ann Benoit
Marjolijn Bijlefeld
Kathryn Black
Connie Boggan
Rebecca Broderick
Marianne Brorup-Weston
Darla Buchacher
Teresa Christensen
Margaret Cleghorn
Dina Conte
Jocelyn Conway
Pamela Cooper
Denise Coursen
Debby Crail
Marlene Cullen
Cathy Daub
Gabriela Oria de Quiñzanos
Holly Derheim
Donna Drozd
Juli Duncan

Janeen Earwood
Judy Elder
Ingrid Enriquez
Trish Evans
Kathleen Gray Farthing
Nancy Ferrato
Michele Fletcher
Meryl Foster
Joanne Frazer
Erica Ginter
Linda Gioia
Miriam Giskin
Alexandra Gruber-Malkin
Chris Gurniak
Hygeia Halfmoon
Kate Hallberg
Elizabeth Handler
Leslie Haynes and Jay Eirling
Nancy Herzog
Mary Heugel
Lynelle Hofman
Michelle Holman
Mary Honas
Rhonda Howard
Linda Howes

Susan Huntley
Caroline Huntress
Beth Irikura
Margaret Cahill Kampa
Helen Kimball-Brooke
Paula Klima
April Kubachka
Leanne Labreche
Jill Langer
Kathryn Leatherwood
Kelly Lewis
Corey Lie-Nielsen
Lorie Lifrieri
Lori Lloyd
Tammy Madkins
Chris McAllister
Kathy McDonald
Kathy Meier
Hope Melnick
Diane Hatzepetros Middleton
Nina Miller
Kristin Minor
Jennifer Monn
Catherine Nicholson
Anne Notarpietro
Wendi Oldham

Wendy Oliver
Heidi Osusky
JoAnna Parente
Shannon Pennington
Kari Pessarra
Monica Sue Petkac
Beth Pirkle
Bunny Poguette
Susan Pollard
Toni Rakestraw
Katie Ritts
Nellie Sabin
Jamie Schluessel

Mary Jean Schweiter-
  Lowe
Mary Short
Heidi Spinelli
Jennifer Steward
Kathryn Stonehocker
Fae Stuart
Sheila Stubbs
Jamie Swann
Jane Szczepaniak
Lucy Till
Sunday Tortelli
Raven Noel Twichell

Michelle Varney
Karin Virnig
Pamela Vollans-
  Matthews
Karen Vradelis
Megan Weeks
Lisa Wilberding
Susan Will
Mary Wilson
Denise Woods
Regina Wootner
Janene Yokoyama
Cindy Zimmerman

Introduction

BE THANKFUL you're having your VBAC today. Although VBACs—it stands for vaginal birth after cesarean and is pronounced "vee-back"—have been occurring all over the United States in tiny numbers for most of this century, the medical profession now welcomes VBACs with unprecedented enthusiasm. In 1995 (the latest available year), 35.5 percent of U.S. women who had previously given birth by cesarean had vaginal births subsequently—almost six times the rate of the previous decade. And the number of VBACs in this country keeps climbing, pushed upward by some combination of medical research, consumer desire, and insurance company directives.

A Brief History of Cesareans and VBACs

For the past seventy years, the adage "Once a cesarean, always a cesarean" has dominated childbirth practices in this country, for several reasons. First of all, not many cesareans took place for most of this seventy-year period (in 1965 the U.S. cesarean rate was 4.5 percent, for example, as compared to 24.7 percent in 1988), and doctors tended to perform them only in dire circumstances. An "unnecessary" cesarean was unimaginable years ago. In addition, until the 1980s cesareans were often performed with the classical "up-and-down" incision, from the belly button down to the pubic bone. Even today this type of incision scar is considered incompatible with a VBAC, because of concerns that a scar of this type could rupture more easily during the hard contractions of labor. Since the mid-1980s, 99 percent of cesarean scars are of the VBAC-friendly, side-to-side lower incision type known as the "bikini cut."

Until the 1980s researchers showed little interest in studying the outcomes of VBACs. The number of cesareans done today—more than 800,000 a year, which is a fourfold increase over thirty years—has been a real attention getter, especially at a time when governmental and medical groups say there are too many surgical births.

The outcome for a woman and her newborn is usually better after a VBAC than a repeat cesarean, as hundreds of VBAC studies have shown. Encouraged by this positive trend, managed-care insurance companies—health maintenance organizations (HMOs) and preferred provider organizations (PPOs) in particular—have served to increase the number of VBACs by actively encouraging vaginal births and even on occasion refusing to pay for elective (i.e., not medically necessary) repeat cesareans. And, for at least two decades, an added catalyst for more VBACs has been consumer interest, led by persistent VBAC pioneers, both childbirth activists and healthcare providers.

Why I Wrote This Book

My job is not to persuade a woman who wants a repeat cesarean to have a VBAC. Instead, my challenge is to show those of you who do want a VBAC how to get one. This book will give you information about what helps and what hinders, guidelines on what to expect, and VBAC stories written in women's own words.

Having a VBAC is not exactly the same as "just" having a vaginal birth. You need to look at the big picture. First of all, it's important that you know why you had your cesarean(s) and what you can do differently next time in order to have a vaginal birth. It's also essential that you understand and appreciate your feelings about giving birth. Armed with sound information and moral support—and with no true contraindications for a vaginal birth—the odds are good that you will have a VBAC this time around.

Unlike most of you, I had my four children in the 1960s, a time when having a cesarean was a rarity, so I've had neither a cesarean nor a VBAC. In writing this book, then, I've relied on more than one hundred women who sent me their VBAC stories, on published research from around the world, and on the lessons I've learned from writing about pregnancy and birth over the past twenty years.

The VBAC Letters

Of all birth stories, VBAC stories in particular radiate triumph and accomplishment, heart and emotion. The vast majority of these letters came from mothers who had VBACs (the exception being a dad who wrote about his wife's labor assistant). I've also included letters from mothers who attempted vaginal birth but who, for various reasons, delivered by cesarean. They are full of just as much feeling and effort as the other stories, and serve to remind us that no one can be guaranteed a 100 percent success rate.

The women who sent these letters live in thirty-two states, plus an American living in the Philippines and two women in the U.S. military. These VBAC babies were born in hospitals, birth centers, homes, and even one in the car on the way to the hospital. Ohio and Washington had the most respondents; nearly a dozen came from Canada, four from England, and one each from Mexico and Australia. All of the writers' names are listed in the Acknowledgments.

The letters reflect a sign of changing times, the trend of more women to use midwives and birth assistants (also called doulas or labor assistants). About one-fourth of the writers had a cesarean for a supposed cephalopelvic disproportion, or CPD (when the baby's head is too big for the birth canal), yet with rare exception, subsequent babies born vaginally to these women were larger, ranging from one-half to two pounds heavier. Three out of four writers had one cesarean before their VBAC; the rest had two or more, and one woman who now lives in Idaho had seven cesareans before she had an uneventful hospital VBAC in Illinois. Three sets of twins were born by VBAC. Most women who wrote in had one VBAC, although some had two or more. The woman who traveled the farthest was a mother in Juneau, Alaska—where VBACs weren't permitted for homebirths—who traveled eighteen hundred miles to a midwife in Eugene, Oregon, in the 1990s.

In my requests for stories, I asked women to describe what person or factor was the most helpful to them in getting a VBAC. Twenty-two books were mentioned, the most popular being *Silent Knife,* by Nancy Wainer Cohen and Lois Estner, followed by *A Good Birth, A Safe Birth,* which I co-authored with Roberta M. Scaer. Helpful doctors and midwives receive enthusiastic praise, as do husbands or partners, and hospital-based and independent childbirth classes. (Those mentioned by name are Birth Works, the Bradley Method, and ALACE—all are in the Resource Directory.) But the most VBAC-helpful person, if measured by times mentioned, is the birth assistant.

I've included as many stories as possible, and I apologize that space considerations prevented me from including more. My desire is that these excerpts from women's letters offer you hope for your own VBAC, strength to persevere, and information to help you get what you want.

What's in This Book

Chapter 1 describes the many advantages of a VBAC over an elective cesarean for both you and your baby. It also includes information about cesareans and VBACs in other countries. Chapter 2 describes women's common fears about VBAC and suggests ways to cope with these fears. Planning your VBAC based on your cesarean history is covered in Chapter 3, followed in Chapter 4 by a description of common insurance options and ways to get the most out of your coverage. Chapters 5 and 6 give tips on the two most critical issues in having a VBAC: finding a VBAC-friendly doctor or midwife and hospital or birth center. Chapter 7 provides information about your other helpers—your partner, labor assistant, and childbirth educator, as well as supportive VBAC organizations.

Everything you need to know about having a VBAC labor is in Chapter 8. Chapter 9 focuses on appreciating your birth experience, with all of its surprises—whether you have a VBAC or another cesarean—and includes information on how to plan the "ideal" cesarean.

Appendix A contains charts of VBAC, cesarean, and infant mortality statistics from other countries so that you can see how the United States measures up. Appendix B is a Resource Directory, which lists helpful organizations and provides phone and fax numbers and e-mail addresses. (Many of these groups will give referrals to support hotlines, healthcare providers, and publications.) The Bibliographic References detail the publications on which my information is based. In case you would like to send me your VBAC story, comments, or questions, a questionnaire appears at the back of the book.

❧ ❧ ❧

A Note on Gender: Because the enrollment of women in medical schools has increased fourfold in the past twenty-five years, and because virtually all midwives, nearly all nurses, and most obstetrical residents are now women, I've used female pronouns throughout this book when referring to medical providers.

And one last comment: Take only what you want from this book, and ignore the rest.

PART ONE

Understanding

CHAPTER 1

🌿 🌿 🌿

Have a VBAC—Here's Why

Cesareans and VBACs Around the World
What Doctors Say About VBACs
Advantages for Babies Born by VBAC
Advantages for Mothers Who Have VBACs

YOU HAVE had a cesarean—maybe even more than one. Perhaps you are already convinced you will have a vaginal birth the next time, or maybe you're only starting to think about a VBAC.

Although there will always be excellent medical reasons for cesareans, repeat cesareans are no longer regarded as a necessity. Some women and their physicians believe that many babies are better off if they're born by surgery, especially if the woman has had a previous cesarean. This belief is due in part to the U.S. infant mortality rate, which has dropped at the same time the cesarean rate has increased.

But the falling infant mortality rate and the increased cesarean rate are not actually linked. Public health researchers say fewer babies die in the developed world today not because of more cesareans, but rather due to improved neonatal care, better birth control, legal abortion, prenatal care, blood banks, and clean water supply, among other reasons.

Cesareans and VBACs Around the World

A nation's infant mortality rate—that is, the number of babies who die in their first year per 1,000 live births—is the gold standard for the country's health. The United States ranks twenty-second in the world in infant mortality, even though it outspends the first twenty-one countries in maternity care and newborn costs. More babies survive per capita in Japan than in any other country; its infant mortality rate is nearly twice as good as ours (4.2 percent, versus 8 percent for the United States, in 1994) and its cesarean rate is half of ours (11.2 percent, versus 20.8 percent for the United States, in 1995).

Many U.S. writers on childbirth, myself included, have written that most European women who have had cesareans have VBACs the second time around. After corresponding with healthcare statisticians on five continents, I can't document this claim. Most countries, in fact, don't keep track of their VBAC rates. In those countries that have kept track, in both Europe and Asia, VBAC rates are indeed higher than in the United States, but (as you can see in the chart on page 180) these European rates are still only around 50 percent. Throughout the developed world, then, repeat cesareans are still more common than VBACS, although the VBAC rate is rising in all of the countries that track it.

The cesarean rate is falling in the United States, Canada, and Australia, but in many countries it's still going up. Brazil (75 percent cesarean rate in urban private clinics and 38 percent in urban public hospitals for 1994), Chile (36 percent in the 1990s), and some other Latin American countries have always performed more cesareans than the United States has. And in 1995 Singapore (27 percent), Portugal (24.3 percent), and Italy (22.4 percent) were ahead of the United States (20.8 percent) in their cesarean rates, too.

Women in Latin American countries who want cesareans give several reasons for their preference. They fear labor and want the convenience of scheduling a birth. They also want to avoid a "stretched vagina," and they believe vaginal births require later surgical repair. However, because a woman's body goes through many changes in readiness for childbirth, it's unlikely that any woman's vagina is the same as it was before she gave birth, regardless of the method. The vagina, or birth canal, aided by hormones that naturally soften and expand the tissues, stretches as the baby emerges in a vaginal birth. Typically, a woman's vagina returns to a firm and taut state after childbirth.

Another reason why women ask for cesareans in Brazil in particular is that having a surgical birth is the easiest way to get a tubal ligation. (An estimated 80 percent of all tubal ligations in Brazil occur during the repair after a cesarean.) In Brazil a tubal ligation is difficult to obtain through the appropriate channels; but when it is performed during a cesarean, the words "tubal ligation" apparently don't appear on any hospital paperwork. Despite what Brazilian women believe to be the advantages that cesareans provide, the Brazilian maternal mortality rate (an estimated 200 deaths per 100,000 births) is more than twenty times that of women in the United States. It is believed that the frequent use of birth technology in less than ideal circumstances plays a role in this high rate.

In some countries, getting a VBAC can put a woman at risk of having her children removed from her care. Three British women were threatened with legal action by their local Social Services departments in the 1990s because they had had VBACs in hospitals outside of the departments' jurisdiction instead of having repeat cesareans at nearby hospitals. In all three cases—in one of them the mother was actually labeled "educationally backward"—the mothers were found in court to be in the right.

In commenting on the cultural differences surrounding childbirth, the French surgeon and childbirth pioneer Michel Odent, who now works in London, posed the following questions: "Why do a majority of French women have a planned epidural birth [see section on epidurals on page 152], yet Moroccan women living in Orléans, France, want a natural birth because a woman in their culture who has not given birth vaginally is not regarded as a real woman? Why do 98 percent of Swedish women want to breastfeed versus 42 percent of French women? Why are painkillers in general and epidural anesthesia in particular rarely used in Japan, one of the most technologically advanced countries?"

Not only do differences exist in childbirth statistics by country, but differences exist within our own country as well. In the United States, cesarean, VBAC, breastfeeding, and infant mortality rates vary by region and by state. VBACs, for example, occur most in the West (36.5 percent) and least in the South (26.0 percent).

The financial aspect of cesarean birth also cannot be discounted. For some time, research has shown that in the United States women who have private insurance and who are past the age of thirty, and especially thirty-five, are more likely to have cesareans. That's true in some other countries as well: private insurance is a known factor in the high cesarean rates in Italy, Brazil, and Singapore.

Other factors that contribute to U.S. cesareans—the use of electronic fetal monitoring, malpractice fears (see page 90), elective inductions, and scheduling convenience—are playing a part in the increasing cesarean rates in other countries, too. The maternity units in Denmark that used electronic fetal monitors, for example, showed a 15 percent higher unplanned cesarean rate than those that used hand-held fetoscopes. In Finland, the risk of having a cesarean was one-and-a-half times greater when labor induction was elective.

What Doctors Say About VBACs

Today the American College of Obstetricians and Gynecologists strongly urges its members to counsel and encourage women to plan labor rather than schedule a repeat surgery. Based on current evidence, almost all women with prior cesareans can plan a VBAC, including women with two or more lower uterine incisions, women who had a prior cesarean due to failure to progress or cephalopelvic disproportion (or CPD, when the baby's head is too big for the birth canal), non-diabetic women expecting a baby weighing more than 4,000 grams (8 pounds, 13 ounces), or women who plan to use an epidural, Pitocin, and/or prostaglandin gel.

The American Academy of Family Physicians holds the belief that a trial of labor after a previous low transverse cesarean section, in the absence of ongoing contraindications, is safe for most women. The AAFP conducted a comprehensive review and meta-analysis of the literature to determine outcomes, costs, and women's preferences by method of delivery. About seven out of ten women who undergo a trial of labor after a previous low transverse cesarean section can expect to deliver vaginally. When compared with an elective repeat cesarean section, going through a trial of labor indicates a slightly increased risk of uterine rupture, but a decreased risk of infection, fever, and postpartum bleeding.

Advantages for Babies Born by VBAC

A mountain of research shows that both babies and their mothers benefit from a subsequent vaginal birth. According to the American College of Obstetricians and Gynecologists, the American Academy of Pediatrics, the American Academy of Family Physicians, and midwives everywhere, babies are healthier, mothers have fewer problems, and both go home sooner from the hospital after vaginal births.

Babies born vaginally are usually born when they are ready, rather than prematurely by surgery. On average, babies born by cesarean have lower birth weights and have completed fewer weeks of gestation than vaginally born babies, which suggests that many cesareans occur before labor begins. These babies account for the majority of admissions to high-risk nurseries. Although some of them are born before their due dates because of medical emergencies that threatened their safety or the safety of their mothers, others are probably born too soon because labor was induced or because the cesarean was scheduled ahead of time, according to a miscalculated due date. These problems are less frequent with cesareans performed after labor begins naturally.

> ❧ *They took my second child too early. After amniocentesis, to see if his lungs were ready to be born, they took him the next day. It wasn't until after I had him and he was very small and very sickly that I realized that they performed the cesarean in his thirty-sixth week. So he was a whole month early and definitely not ready. He's had a lifetime of illness and sickness as a result of it.*
>
> *— Jodi B., Indiana*

Babies born through the birth canal have the benefit of a surge of the hormones called catecholamines, which are essential for survival. These hormones, one of which is adrenaline, are found in much higher levels in vaginally born babies. Catecholamines are secreted by

🍂 Advantages for Babies Born by VBAC

* Babies born vaginally are usually born when they are ready.
* Babies born through the birth canal have the benefit of a cate-cholamine surge.
* Babies born through the birth canal are much more likely to be born with healthy lungs.
* Babies born vaginally have higher Apgar scores.
* Babies born through the birth canal enjoy early, frequent contact with their mothers.
* Babies born vaginally are much more likely to be breastfed.

the infant's adrenal glands, which lie above the kidneys and are released in the baby in high amounts during labor, sometimes changing the fetal heart rate. They prepare the infant for survival outside the womb. They help to clear the infant's lungs in preparation for normal breathing, speed up his metabolic rate for quick stabilization, and promote a rich supply of blood to his heart and brain. The catecholamine surge of a vaginally born baby keeps a newborn alert for some time. These hormones also dilate the pupils of his eyes, probably in preparation for the "falling in love" bonding that takes place at birth between a newborn and his parents.

This doesn't mean that cesarean-born babies are never alert or don't experience "falling in love" bonding with their parents. What is true, though, is that babies born vaginally experience mechanical advantages of coming through the birth canal (the natural squeeze that puts pressure on the baby's chest to push fluid out of the lungs, esophagus, nose, and throat), which give them the highest levels on average of the hormonal surge. Babies who are born by cesarean but experience some labor prior to surgery are in the medium range of these catecholamine levels, while babies who are born by scheduled cesarean with no prior labor have the lowest amounts of this circulating hormone.

Babies born through the birth canal are much more likely to be born

with healthy lungs. Respiratory distress syndrome, sometimes known as hyaline membrane disease, is a condition in which the baby's lungs are not strong enough to get sufficient oxygen to body tissues. This problem, which is aggravated by anesthesia (in particular general anesthesia) and lower levels of catecholamines, is twenty times more likely to occur in babies born by cesarean prior to the onset of labor. In addition, these babies are more likely to be put on mechanical ventilators in neonatal intensive care nurseries than infants with other respiratory illnesses.

> ✍ Jon's cesarean was no less traumatic than my first. Jon was delivered to his parents' delight and joy—a boy! But Jon was a blue-gray color. They gave me a brief cheek stroke—his to mine, since I was strapped down—and rushed him off. The nightmare began. It seemed he had fluid in his lungs. I wasn't allowed to hold, touch, or see him except through a window for four days!
>
> —Cindy Z., Pennsylvania

Babies born vaginally have higher Apgar scores. An Apgar is a means of assessing the health status of a newborn at intervals of 1 and 5 minutes after birth. It measures, in scores that range from 0 to 10, heart rate, breathing, muscle tone, response to stimuli, and skin color. Of course it makes sense that a baby in distress that needs to be delivered by cesarean might have a lower Apgar score—especially one born to a woman who had (rarely used) general anesthesia instead of regional anesthesia. In a 1995 study of uncomplicated, full-term pregnancies, most babies regardless of how they were born did not require nursery stays or breathing support. However, when the 10,871 vaginally born babies were compared to those 538 infants born by elective cesarean because of CPD or "failure to progress," there were marked differences. The surgically born babies were more likely to need intermediate or intensive care at birth along with respiratory support, and were more likely to have 1-minute Apgar scores of less than 4.

Babies born through the birth canal enjoy early, frequent contact with their mothers. A woman who has a cesarean often gets only a glimpse of her baby immediately after birth. Sometimes a baby is taken away quickly to be checked, in part, because he may have a higher risk for a number of newborn problems. The mother will remain in the operating room to have her incision sewn up, and then move on to a surgical recovery area. A woman who gives birth vaginally, on the other hand, can eat, drink, and move around as well as feed and care for her newborn immediately, if she so desires. When a VBAC mom takes her baby home, she's much more likely to be able to give her newborn more of her attention, because she is not recovering from surgery and does not have the accompanying postoperative pain.

> ✐ *Happily, my baby boy who was born by cesarean was healthy, but a number of complications arose for me, and I was hospitalized for nearly five days and felt totally exhausted and weak. My baby, under observation for twenty-four hours, was not allowed out of the nursery and was given a bottle despite our protests. He became nipple-confused and our breastfeeding got off to a rocky and challenging start. Even after I made it home, my recovery seemed incredibly slow and I felt uncomfortable and unlike myself for a very long time. Needless to say, while I was delighted with my baby, and would have gone through the experience all over again if I had to just to have him, I could not help but wonder if all that trauma to my body and my spirit could have been avoided.*
>
> *Four years later my husband and I revelled in the whole magical experience of natural childbirth with the birth of our second child, which was healing in ways for both of us. Surrounded by supportive and helpful friends in the comfort of my own bed, I was amazed at how healthy and well I actually felt. As for breastfeeding, my daughter latched on easily, with none of the difficulties I had experienced with my son. Today, my baby is nine weeks old, and I am completely recovered physically and spiritually. I am at peace with the experience of my son's birth, thrilled with my VBAC, and will be forever grateful that I have these two healthy and incredible children, however they came into the world.*
>
> *—Patience A., Wisconsin*

Babies born vaginally are much more likely to be breastfed and to be nursed for a longer time span. The first days of a baby's life are critical to breastfeeding success, and successful breastfeeding is easiest when the early stimulation of the breast created by the baby's sucking produces a bountiful milk supply. Giving birth vaginally makes this process much easier. For example, when babies are with their mothers uninterrupted for the first hour after birth, after twenty minutes or so most infants will begin rooting motions and, if given the opportunity, will make crawling movements toward the breast in an effort to latch on. Likewise, babies who "room in" with their mothers from birth, and who nurse at will, gain more weight and nurse well sooner, on average. Off to a good start, these are the same babies who probably will nurse for more months overall.

It's no surprise, then, that mothers who have cesareans, especially emergency surgeries or cesareans with general anesthesia, are less successful in getting breastfeeding started. Around the world, women who are coping with the consequences of surgery, including delayed recovery, have more difficulty getting breastfeeding established. Even those women who are highly committed to breastfeeding, and who eventually nurse for many months, can experience delays, sometimes for days, in nursing their infants after a cesarean delivery.

> *After Rod was born, they held him up to me to see, but I could not hold him—my husband could. I went to recovery, and forty-five minutes later I held him for the first time in my room, but I was not allowed to sit up for twelve hours because of the spinal. I nursed him on one side, then called for a nurse to turn me to the other side because I was still numb. That was my cesarean. My second child, Ruby, was born [vaginally] six years later. She was 7 pounds, 12 ounces, screaming and healthy. What a difference! Ruby nursed right away and really clamped on!*
>
> —*Jennifer M., Pennsylvania*

> *My first child, Ian, was born via cesarean section for failure to progress and CPD. I had been in labor for fifteen hours, and had been receiving Pitocin for ten of those hours. I was at 3 centimeters and the doctor decided a cesarean was indicated. The surgery was frightening, and my postpartum period was very long and difficult. I had a negative reaction to all the pain medication given to me in the hospital and I was very sick for the first several weeks after Ian was born. Because of this I was unable to successfully breastfeed and suffered through postpartum depression for months afterwards. Anna [her child born by VBAC] took instantly to*

breastfeeding. I had no postpartum complications, no depression, and Anna is still breastfeeding as she nears her second birthday.

—*Lynelle H., Washington*

Advantages for Mothers Who Have VBACs

With a VBAC, the risk for infection after the birth drops from as high as 35 percent (with a cesarean) down to 2 to 4 percent. Different hospitals and researchers report varying infection rates associated with cesarean births, with and without the use of antibiotics. Typically, the use of antibiotics before surgery reduces the infection rate, but, unfortunately, antibiotics are not always effective. In addition, some post-cesarean infections don't show up until a mother has gone home—a particular concern given today's shorter hospital stays. Infections that occur after mothers have left the hospital are unlikely to show up in studies because most researchers gather information from women's hospital records alone.

One of the two most common infections after a cesarean is endometritis, an infection of the lining of the uterus that causes fever and abdominal tenderness. Who gets this infection is based on a number of factors. The number of vaginal exams you had before surgery

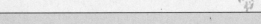

◢ Advantages for Mothers Who Have VBACs

- The risk for infection after the birth drops from as high as 35 percent down to 2 to 4 percent.
- Other surgical hazards decrease, including extra blood loss, the need for blood transfusions, urinary tract damage, and placental disorders.
- Women recover more quickly, sometimes by many months.
- Women do not experience cesarean depression.
- Women feel more attached to their babies sooner.
- The parents will probably save on medical costs.

can play a part in your susceptibility to infection: half of the women who have six or more vaginal exams develop endometritis despite the use of preventive antibiotics. Other factors that increase your risk for infection are your physician's skill and experience, your choice of hospital, how long your membranes were broken before the birth, or if you were sick before you went into labor.

The risk for endometritis is higher for women who have bacterial vaginosis, also known as vaginitis, a common vaginal infection. Insulin-dependent women who receive antibiotics immediately before or after the cesarean are also at a higher risk, as are women who have a planned cesarean (either primary or repeat) or who have their cesareans before twenty-eight weeks of gestation. Women who are at greatest risk for endometritis after a cesarean are teenagers and women who are poor—probably because most of them receive little or no prenatal care—as well as women who had been connected to an internal fetal monitor prior to surgery.

A wound infection is also common after a cesarean. You are most likely to contract this if you had ruptured membranes longer than six hours before the birth, if you were connected to an internal fetal monitor, or if you were either double your normal body weight or a hundred pounds over your normal weight at the birth, which would make it difficult to stitch together the layers of the abdomen. Other risks related to cesarean surgery include a return to the hospital for repairs, along with a risk for abscess, peritonitis, gangrene, urinary tract damage, and placental disorders. As with any other major abdominal operation, surgery opens up a higher risk for hemorrhage, and as many as 10 percent of the women who have cesareans need blood transfusions. The average blood loss from a vaginal birth is about a pint; from a cesarean, almost a quart.

Other possible surgical consequences are a temporary paralysis of the bladder and bowel, a hysterectomy, a retained piece of the placenta (which occasionally happens after a vaginal birth, too), or a surgical item left in your body, which will require follow-up surgery. An infrequent injury, but one that is three times more likely to occur after a repeat cesarean than a first cesarean, is urinary tract damage associated with dense bladder adhesions from the first surgery.

❧ Three weeks after Liam's birth, I was admitted into the hospital with a major uterine infection. A piece of placenta had been left behind. I was separated from Liam for three days. It was a very traumatic time for both of us, and nursing him was hard to reestablish after that. After repeated infections that no amount of drugs would clear up, I had to stop nursing to take a combination of three antibiotics for a month. This finally did fix the problem. I was feeling very bitter, and at this point I didn't know whether I could even conceive again.

—Wendy A., Quebec, Canada

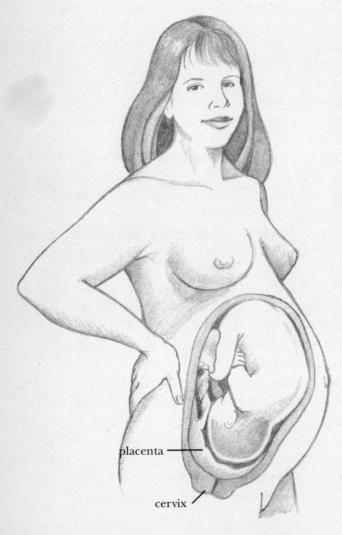

placenta ——

cervix

Placenta previa. This is a condition in which the placenta covers the cervix (usually, the placenta attaches high on the uterine wall). In the illustration, the placenta completely covers the cervix, blocking the entrance to the vagina. When this happens— usually in the last trimester—the mother bleeds painlessly and may need blood transfusions. She must have a cesarean.

Sometimes the placenta only partially covers the cervix. In this case, if it's too early for the baby to be born, the mother stays in bed until all bleeding stops. She may be able to give birth vaginally.

Placenta previa occurs in about 1 in 200 pregnancies. However, the risk increases two to five times for a woman who has had a prior cesarean.

Placenta accreta. This is a condition in which part or all of the placenta adheres abnormally to the uterine wall. The placenta actually invades the muscular layer of the uterine wall, because the layer that's supposed to be there, the decidua, is poorly formed. Placenta accreta often occurs along with placenta previa. Massive hemorrhage is common with placenta accreta, and usually *results in the woman having a hysterectomy. The baby is usually affected as well.*

Placenta accreta is most likely to occur in women who have had uterine surgery. The risk increases with each cesarean incision. This is because scarred uterine tissue can interfere with the normal process of a low-implanted placenta moving away from the cervix as the uterus expands.

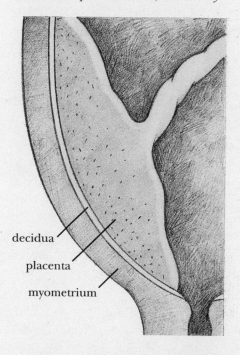

decidua

placenta

myometrium

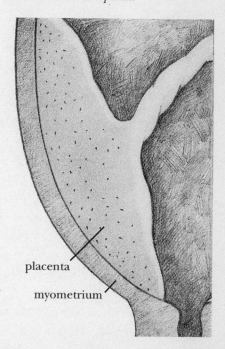

placenta

myometrium

The chances of developing dangerous placental problems during pregnancy, such as placenta previa (the placenta covers the birth canal opening) and placenta accreta (the placenta grows into the wall of the uterus), increase significantly with a woman's subsequent cesareans. Sometimes this happens because the surgeon makes a new uterine incision rather than cutting open the old scar. In this case, although a woman may have only one visible scar on her abdomen from all her surgeries, her uterus will have one uterine scar per cesarean. Each of these placental disorders occurs at least two to three times more often than uterine rupture occurs in VBACs.

The ultimate cesarean tragedy, of course, is a rare one: the death of the mother after childbirth. Women who have cesareans are two to four times more likely to die after childbirth than women who give birth vaginally. Many of those who die, it should be noted, are categorized as high-risk during pregnancy or develop unusual problems during childbirth. In 1993, at least 302 U.S. women died out of the nearly 4 million women who gave birth (the National Center for Health Statistics and other researchers estimate that because of poor reporting this number might be three times higher). Among the leading causes for maternal death are hemorrhage, complications resulting from general anesthesia, hypertensive disorders, infections, and pulmonary embolisms. There have been no published reports of a healthy woman dying after a uterine rupture that occurred while she attempted a VBAC in a hospital.

Two large-scale studies have compared the maternal risk of having an elective cesarean with that of attempting a VBAC. A Canadian study comparing 3,249 women who attempted VBACs with 2,889 women who had elective cesareans made the headlines in 1996. Most of the attention was probably due to the authors' statement that "major" maternal complications occurred twice as often with the attempted VBACs. A careful reading of the report, however, shows that the words *major* and *minor* are applied in ways that most physicians would dispute. For example, blood transfusions and wound infections, which occurred more frequently with women who had elective cesareans, are labeled minor. Regardless of the "major" and "minor" labels, the two groups of women had comparable outcomes.

Another large-scale study, performed in California in 1994, found fairly similar outcomes in women who attempted VBACS and others who had elective cesareans. But the group of 2,207 mothers who had elective cesareans had longer hospital stays, more fevers, and more transfusions than the group of 5,022 women who had VBACs.

Of course complications can and do occur with vaginal births. However, if you compare a "routine" cesarean with an uncomplicated vaginal childbirth, it's safe to say that the risk for complications increases with surgical birth.

Women who give birth vaginally recover more quickly, sometimes by many months. Although some medical literature suggests that recovery from a cesarean should take only four weeks, that's not what many women say. One study reported that six weeks after the birth about one-third of women who had cesareans had regained their usual energy, while three-fourths of the women who gave birth vaginally had done so by that time.

Other research shows that at least one-fourth of women who had cesareans were still not fully recovered at six months post partum, and most found the recovery period to be much more difficult than they had anticipated. The easier recovery from a vaginal birth is a boon for any woman caring for an infant, especially for a woman who has other small children or who is returning to a job outside the home. Women typically return to their jobs in the workplace within eight weeks of the birth.

I could not believe the recovery time after my VBAC. I was fairly well recovered by one week post partum, and by two weeks I felt as if I'd never been pregnant. Rebecca has been an easy baby from the beginning, and I believe that the early cuddling and nursing have helped to shape her personality. She has not been out of my sight ever; even in the hospital they brought the bilirubin lights right into my room. I have been driving, picking up my older daughter Barbara and holding Rebecca, and functioning as a normal person from my first day home. It has been amazing! There is no comparison to my first birth.

—Regina W., Colorado

I was so thankful for the opportunity to deliver vaginally. For me, the episiotomy stitches didn't recover quicker than my abdominal ones—my bottom was very sore for a while—but I had so much more energy, and could actually go without sleep and look forward to waking up with Drew in the middle of the night just to be alone with him. With Jacob, who was born by cesarean, I thought I felt good and recovered great, but the exhaustion didn't leave for probably six months. I think that is the best aspect of a VBAC—that you recover so much easier, which helps with other children around.

—Wendi O., Georgia

❧ The biggest benefit of the VBAC, aside from the actual birth experience, was that sex, which had been painful ever since the cesarean birth of our son, stopped hurting. I read somewhere later that this is not an uncommon phenomenon. Apparently when scar tissue or healing from a first birth isn't quite right, the passage of the second baby through the birth canal serves to stretch or break the adhesions that may have been causing pain. What can I say? It worked for me.

—Beth P., California

Women who give birth vaginally do not experience cesarean depression, which sometimes lasts for many months. Nearly all women experience the so-called "baby blues," if only for a few days or a few weeks after childbirth; postpartum blues occur when the normal hormonal changes in a woman's body combine with lack of sleep and a temporary reaction to some drugs used during childbirth. The up-and-down feelings that come after a vaginal birth seldom last long, in part because women who have vaginal births do not have the physical debilitation that surgery often creates.

Cesarean depression, on the other hand, which as many as 40 percent of women who have had cesareans may experience, packs more of a punch for several reasons. A woman who has had a cesarean is recovering from major surgery, and like all post-surgical patients she requires extra bed rest and special attention paid to incision pain and other post-surgical changes. Add to this burden the fact that a woman who has had a cesarean is also a new mother, who needs to care for an infant twenty-four hours a day. This new mother may also have other small children, which adds to her workload—one that is much more manageable after a vaginal birth.

Cesarean depression features some of the same elements that lead to the baby blues or postpartum depression except that the post-cesarean mom needs more rest and may be more likely to react to the medication used during childbirth. A surgical birth of course requires more drugs than a vaginal one, as well as drug use for days afterward to relieve surgical pain, and sometimes this combination of drugs can produce negative side effects.

Women who have had cesareans are less able to handle the challenges an infant presents because they are physically weakened and, perhaps, emotionally distressed as well. A woman who has had a cesarean often is dealing with other issues that can play a role in her depression, among them a sense of failure and disappointment that lasts for six months or so. Women who have emergency cesareans experience a sixfold higher incidence of depression. Negative feelings such as these may last many months, even years.

🌿 *The incredible joy and wonder a new baby brings was there, but there was also disappointment and sadness that once again instead of giving birth, my baby had been surgically removed from my body. Often cesarean parents are discouraged from grieving for the losses they've experienced by reproofs such as, "You have a healthy baby, what more do you want?" But it's normal to mourn the loss of hopes and dreams of a peaceful vaginal birth. Birth is important! I had planned for this birth for so long and had put so much effort into it, it just didn't seem fair I ended up having another cesarean. For a while I just wanted to enjoy my baby and not think about the disappointment of her birth. I didn't want her first days and weeks to be filled with a sad, crying mother, because I really was very happy with her and with having a baby in our family. So for a while I just enjoyed her and didn't think much about the birth. After a while I could start to deal with some of the negative feelings I had about the birth. Mostly I felt betrayed by my body. I was angry because I felt I'd done "all the right things" and yet had ended up with a cesarean. I felt if only I'd done some things differently during labor, then things would not have happened the way they did.*

—Kelly L., Virginia

If you've wondered why you did or didn't experience cesarean depression, you may find illuminating two contrasting profiles that have emerged from research on new mothers' expectations, beliefs, and experiences. Perhaps you'll find a little of yourself in both lists, but chances are that one profile fits you best.

The women who are *most* likely to experience cesarean depression are those who:

- *Expected natural childbirth.* You wanted not only a vaginal birth, but dreamed of an unmedicated childbirth. Perhaps you planned to give birth in the hospital's low-tech birthing room, or you started labor at an out-of-hospital birth center or at home. The last thing you expected was a cesarean.

- *May have had inadequate help and support during the cesarean and/or after the surgery.* Perhaps your partner was not permitted or unavailable to be with you during surgery, and no one else was with you, either. Women need to discuss their children's births, and this may prove difficult unless someone else in the operating room can tell you what happened in great detail later. While you were in the hospital, you probably didn't have friends and family available to help you hold or breastfeed the baby or to help you move around, and hospital nurses may have been so busy with other duties that they couldn't spend much time with you, either. Worst of all, you might have gone home to little or no help—just when you needed it the most.

- *May have had an emergency cesarean, general anesthesia, or a combination of drugs that caused unpleasant, persistent side effects.* An emergency cesarean is an unplanned one, so you weren't prepared for that outcome. With general anesthesia, you were unconscious and unaware of what happened in the operating room, and you didn't know anything about your baby until you awakened in the recovery room. You cannot add up all the possible side effects for one drug—an epidural, for instance—and then add on the possible side effects of another drug—postpartum painkillers—and come up with a complete list of potential problems. When drugs are combined, side effects are not always predictable. Perhaps you were one of those women who is especially sensitive to drug combinations.

- *Felt coerced by the hospital staff and/or by their partner.* Some women rightly or wrongly felt they were pushed into an unnecessary cesarean. One mother still bitterly remembers being at 9 centimeters and being told she needed a cesarean with little explanation for the reasons, while her husband, whom she viewed as her protector, immediately agreed with the hospital staff.

• *Believed that the cesarean was mostly an operation and not a birth experience.* When the hospital staff explains all their actions in advance in a caring manner, which they often do, there are seldom complaints from moms. Unfortunately, that doesn't always happen. Numerous women have said they might as well have had general anesthesia for all the help the operating room staff gave them. Nothing was explained, questions were ignored; and sometimes the only discussion that took place was what the surgeon and nurse were going to have for their next meal.

• *Planned to breastfeed, but found that the aftermath of a cesarean made this too difficult.* This is especially true if your baby had to be separated from you and kept in a nursery, or if you had little or no help in the hospital or at home.

• *Probably experienced complications after surgery or had a difficult convalescence.* It's easy for anyone to feel depressed if you're convalescing longer than anticipated. How much worse might it be if you've been rehospitalized for complications or had an infection?

On the other hand, the women who are *least likely* to experience cesarean depression are those who:

• *Placed a healthy baby ahead of a good birth experience.* The goal was the baby—how he arrived was not the point. If you had had a wonderful birth experience, that would have been an unexpected bonus.

• *Trusted their doctor's judgment and felt their cesarean was necessary.* You not only believed your doctor was right at the time of the cesarean, but even months later, when, typically, some women begin to have doubts, you knew the cesarean was the right thing for you.

- *Planned their cesarean, or knew from the beginning that it was a distinct possibility.* Planning in advance for any surgery always makes for an easier recovery. You probably read books and articles about what happens in a surgical birth, talked to women who had had cesareans, and perhaps took a cesarean class. You also had time to think about and plan for post-surgery needs for you and your newborn instead of worrying about this while you were in the throes of labor.

- *Are not believers in "natural" childbirth and welcome the pain relief of anesthesia.* If you never entertained the idea of a drug-free birth, and always knew immediate pain relief was the logical course for you, you wouldn't be disappointed at all about the medications even if you had some reservations about a surgical birth.

- *May have had other major life events not go according to plan either and thus have learned to adapt.* This is not to say that women who experience cesarean depression can't cope, but those of you who didn't have profound regrets probably had a recovery that met your expectations.

Women who give birth vaginally feel more attached to their babies sooner. Mother-child bonding is an experience that takes a lifetime, but research confirms that the first mother-baby tie can begin mere moments after birth. According to Marshall and Phyllis Klaus and John Kennell, bonding researchers, a healthy newborn will stay awake and alert for forty minutes during his first hour of life and will experience 10 percent of his first week in this intense state.

Women who have VBACs are quick to comment on the differences in their contact with their newborns in the first hours and days in comparison to their post-cesarean experiences. It's true that women who have cesareans can have constant help from family and friends in the hospital, allowing them to spend more time with their newborn than otherwise might have been possible. However, the fatigue and the pain from the surgery makes it difficult, if not impossible, for many of these mothers to hold and feed their babies as much as they would like, and sometimes illness can separate mother and baby.

> *My fifth child was a VBAC. I got to go through the labor and experience it to the end. I touched Anna's head as she descended. I saw her head as she was emerging. I got to feel that blessed sensation just before she totally emerged—the sting and the joy. I got the thrill of pushing and then feeling her come out—such a feeling. The tug and pressure of a c-section has no thrill. There's the excitement of "What will it be?" but you have no control, no involvement. I had my baby fresh from the womb on my belly. I held her and nursed her. No one said nursing should wait until the pediatrician has checked her or until I am more comfortable.*
>
> —Cindy Z., Pennsylvania

With a vaginal birth, the parents will probably save out-of-pocket money because of a shorter hospital stay, no operating-room costs, and fewer drugs and less anesthesia. Between higher physician and hospital birth costs and more and more insurance copayments, few of you will get away without paying something. I'll provide more on this issue in Chapter 4.

❧ ❧ ❧

Whether your cesarean was planned or a surprise, whether you embraced it or found it terrible, whether you had one cesarean or many, you'll find out in the next chapter how to get past any fears you might have about VBAC.

CHAPTER 2

❧ ❧ ❧

Overcome Your Fears of Having a VBAC

Women's Biggest Fears
How to Manage Your VBAC Fears
Why Choose a Repeat Cesarean?
If You Have a History of Childhood Sexual Abuse

VBAC CAN BE a scary idea, but it needn't be. The more information you have, the more reassured—and probably successful—you will be. According to a study published in the *Journal of the American Medical Association,* among many other sources, the women most likely to have VBACs are those who are well informed.

Even if you aren't afraid of having a VBAC, many women are. This chapter describes the most common VBAC fears, and offers ways to help you cope with or triumph over these worries. You'll read why one-third of women who have a history of cesareans refuse VBACs. You'll also get a description of the effects that childhood sexual abuse sometimes has on labor, along with suggestions that have helped women who have such a history.

Women's Biggest Fears

Your fears about having a VBAC might show up at any time—before conception, during the pregnancy, or once labor starts. Women who have VBACs say the fear of going through labor and having another cesarean usually goes away once you get past the stage where you got stuck before, whether that be at 1 centimeter dilation or after four hours of pushing. Those women least likely to worry had vaginal births before their cesareans or had cesareans because their babies were in the breech position. And most women who have VBACs aren't so concerned about the outcome of subsequent births.

Here, then, are women's biggest fears about having a VBAC. Findings from international research on this topic mirror what the women said in the letters I received for this book.

My scar will rupture and my baby will die. This is top on the fear list for many women, and their doctors as well. It is the most serious VBAC risk. Bear in mind, however, that repeat cesareans aren't risk-free either, as pointed out in Chapter 1.

A cesarean requires two incisions, one on the outer skin—that's the scar you can see—and one on the uterus itself. (Sometimes the uterus is sewn up in more than one layer, but there is still only one uterine incision.) These incisions aren't necessarily in the same spot. A uterine incision could be up-and-down, while the incision of the outer skin could be side-to-side.

A uterine "window," or dehiscence, is a symptomless and harmless thinning of the uterine scar tissue. The risk of getting a dehiscence during VBAC is 1 to 2 percent, whether the scar is vertical or horizontal.

Much more dangerous than a dehiscence is a complete uterine rupture. This occurs when the skin of the uterine wall suddenly tears all the way through. When a woman has had a cesarean, any rupture usually occurs in the uterine scar from that surgery, although it can

---

🍃 *Women's Biggest Fears*

• My scar will rupture and my baby will die.
• My body can't labor and give birth like other women's bodies.
• My baby will be too big to get through my birth canal.
• Attempting a VBAC is self-indulgent.
• I fear the unknown, and having another cesarean is a "known."
• I won't be able to stand the pain without medication.
• I will get my hopes up, only to be disappointed.
• The triggers associated with my last cesarean will occur again.

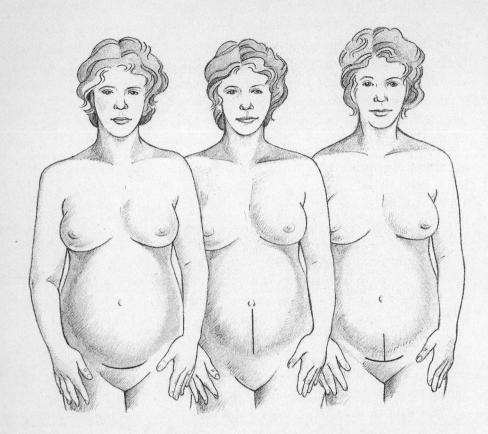

Low-transverse incision, classical incision, and inverted T incision (from left to right). Since the mid-1980s, 99 percent of cesareans have been performed with the low left-to-right horizontal (transverse) incision. This is the safest type, because it is the least likely to rupture. The classical, or vertical, incision was commonly used prior to the 1980s, and is the least VBAC-friendly cesarean incision. Shorter and safer vertical incisions are occasionally used today. The short vertical and the inverted T (a combination short vertical and transverse) incisions are sometimes used for the cesarean delivery of premature babies or for placenta previa (when the placenta is blocking the birth canal), or when the baby is transverse (sideways) in the womb. Current research shows that VBAC is safe with a T or a low vertical incision.

occur elsewhere. Often the only indication of uterine rupture, according to a 1993 study of 106 ruptures in California, is a prolonged slowing of the fetal heart tones. This may be accompanied by excessive blood loss and, if the woman hasn't had anesthesia, abdominal pain.

In the past ten years, 99 percent of cesareans have been performed with the low left-to-right horizontal incision. These are the safest incisions; they are the least likely to rupture because they do less damage to the woman's uterus. Based on the outcomes of many thousands of VBACs, the risk for uterine rupture with a low horizontal scar is about 1 percent. When obstetrician Bruce Flamm—a leading VBAC pioneer—and his colleagues evaluated the VBACs of eleven thousand women in southern California in 1994, the rupture rate was 0.5 percent, or half of 1 percent.

The old-fashioned vertical, or classical, scar has not been studied nearly as often. The estimated rupture rate for this type is 2.2 percent—several times greater than the rupture rate from horizontal scars. Many physicians think it's unsafe for a woman with a classical incision to attempt a VBAC. But some women, after finding a supportive doctor or midwife, do give birth vaginally with a classical incision. One woman from Ohio had an 11-pound baby vaginally with a classical scar.

Recent research shows that VBAC is safe with either an inverted T incision or a low-segment short vertical incision, which is shorter than the classical scar. The short vertical and inverted T incisions are frequently used when a baby is premature or transverse (lying sideways in the womb) and for placenta previa (when the placenta is blocking the birth canal). According to Flamm, data suggest that VBAC is a safe option with the inverted T incision.

❧ I had what is called a "T-cut," and was told that only 1 percent of c-sections are T-cuts and I would never be able to deliver naturally again. My recovery was grueling. I was one of those little old people you see walking aimlessly up and down the halls. Walking was supposed to help; it didn't. During my [third] pregnancy, which was the best one I've had, I tried not to concern myself with the delivery. Three days before my due date, I went into the hospital, and my doctor, who was leaving the next day, ruptured my membranes. When I had my first big contraction, the baby went upward instead of down, leading my doctor to believe that the lining of my uterus was thinning under my breast. At that point the doctor told me that it didn't look like I would be able to do this, and the case room nurse began to prepare me for another c-section. When my bladder emptied, thankfully the baby went downward. After being induced, everything went

well and I delivered the baby vaginally much quicker than everyone thought was possible.

—Diana M., Ontario, Canada

If you are not certain what kind of scar you have, there is still good news. Studies that looked at the VBAC outcomes for women who had unknown scar types show that they did as well as those who had known low horizontal scars.

Ultrasound is sometimes used to determine what kind of scar you have and how likely it is to rupture, but ultrasound has not been a reliable diagnostic tool for this, nor have intrauterine pressure catheters or x-ray pelvimetry. A 1996 French study of 642 women reported on the value of using sonographic measurements at eight months' gestation to measure the thickness of lower uterine segments. It's true that women with the thickest segments didn't have ruptures, but the vast majority of the women with thinner uterine segments didn't have ruptures, either.

The Vaginal Birth After Cesarean Guidelines from the American College of Obstetricians and Gynecologists (ACOG) state that women with two or more cesareans who have low horizontal uterine scars should not be discouraged from having a VBAC. Reports of a VBAC after several cesareans have not been frequent in the medical literature, but several women wrote to me that they had had three or four cesareans—one even had seven cesareans—before they had vaginal births.

Although supported by the ACOG, the use of Pitocin and prostaglandin gel to induce a VBAC labor or the use of Pitocin to speed up a labor has always been controversial. There have been reports of uterine rupture after the use of either Pitocin or gel, especially when they are used in large amounts. A 1997 review of Florida childbirth malpractice claims, for example, showed that seven out of nine uterine ruptures occurred after the use of Pitocin with women whose uteruses were not "ripe," that is, ready for labor. Not all uterine ruptures that occur in labor are associated with these products, however.

A previous cesarean is the usual reason given for a rupture. However, according to the *Cochrane Database of Systematic Reviews,* the largest and most reliable pregnancy and childbirth resource, a history of a cesarean is a factor in less than half of reported cases of uterine rupture. Rupture can occur in any trimester, or in a woman who has not had a cesarean, or even in a woman who is not pregnant. Rupture has occurred, rarely, in all the following situations: after in-vitro fertilization and embryo transfer, after the removal of uterine fibroids using laparoscopy (a procedure in which a thin, lighted instrument is put through a small incision just below the navel), and in laboring women who had a history of dilatation and curettage (D&C).

In the rare instances when complete uterine rupture occurs, serious consequences for the baby are far more common with a vertical scar. There have been instances, however, when a uterine rupture occurred in a woman who had a low horizontal scar, and the result was a baby who either had neurological problems or, in rare cases, died. Consequences for the mother involve additional, and sometimes extreme, blood loss. Uterine ruptures can usually be repaired without a hysterectomy, however.

The risk for uterine rupture is often exaggerated, but it does happen. Because of that, and due to the fact that the best outcome from a rupture for both baby and mother is an immediate cesarean, nearly all doctors and pregnant women who support VBAC are comfortable only if the woman labors in a hospital that is appropriately prepared. (See "Non-Hospital VBACs and the Risk for Uterine Rupture" on page 95.)

My body can't labor and give birth like other women's bodies. Many women who have had cesareans believe this; it's almost as if the experience left that message deep in their cells. Remember that every year around the world hundreds of thousands of women give birth by VBAC. Your body still remembers how to labor and give birth. Your baby—like all babies, if given the opportunity—will start the contractions, working in harmony with the hormones that instigate and maintain labor. It's essential, though, that you work with a doctor or midwife who is convinced that you can have a VBAC.

My baby will be even bigger than the last and won't get through my birth canal. Even if there were a reliable way to estimate a newborn's size—and there isn't—the American College of Obstetricians and Gynecologists claims that the baby's estimated size is not a good indicator of whether a baby can be born vaginally. Of the women who sent me their stories, nearly all who had had cesareans for CPD went on to have bigger babies—ranging from a half-pound to two pounds larger—in subsequent vaginal births.

✒ *I had two main fears about a VBAC. One was the rupture potential, and the other was inadequate pelvic size. As much as I like my doctor— he was the back-up doc for my midwife during my first pregnancy and was very supportive and sensitive through my seven miscarriages—he contributed to my fear of the size of my pelvis. He occasionally referred to my "small" pelvis, even into the last week of my pregnancy. Psychologically, this idea was hard for me to combat. The real surprise came when my son was born vaginally at 7 pounds, 3 ounces, and my daughter born by cesarean weighed only 6 pounds, 6 ounces.*

—Michelle H., Oregon

✒ *I had my daughter by c-section because of her breech position. She weighed 8 pounds, 14 ounces, so there was some concern that I may have to have another c-section if I had another large baby. Four years later I became pregnant. My pregnancy went great and my doctor encouraged me to try a VBAC. To tell the truth I was terrified because I had never experienced labor before. I had asked my doctor if I could choose to have another c-section. He said it was totally up to me and he would support me no matter what I decided. Then he went over all the benefits of a vaginal birth versus a c-section. I had many outsiders offering their opinions on both sides. My husband said it was up to me; he would also support the decision I made. So ultimately it was up to me, and believe me, I was going back and forth up to my thirty-ninth week. We knew the baby was head first, and that this baby would probably be bigger then my daughter was. At my thirty-nine-week visit my doctor said he wanted to induce me the next week. After seven hours of labor I gave birth to my son! I had a successful VBAC, and I'm so happy I did. The amazing part is that my son weighed over 10 pounds!*

—Kari P., Virginia

Attempting a VBAC is self-indulgent. What if I somehow hurt my baby? Whatever the reason for your cesarean, statistically it's not likely to occur again. And even if it does, your expanded knowledge about VBAC and your choice of birth attendant, place of birth, and helpers may alter the outcome this time around. You can develop new ways of working through labor and enlist more people to be on your side.

> 🖉 *As far as worries concerning having a VBAC: yes, I did have some. I didn't want my desire for a natural birth to be a selfish desire. What if I had a very long and hard labor that put stress on the baby? God forbid if something went wrong and the baby was brain damaged or died as a result of the labor. I would never forgive myself. Another worry that became greater as I went past my due date was a fear of failure if I did not succeed in having a VBAC. I had invested a lot of energy and money into trying for a VBAC, and was afraid of potential disappointment. However, I did try to counter that worry with the knowledge that I was doing everything possible to achieve a VBAC, and if I did have to resort to another caesarean, it was because it was essential. In which case, thank goodness for caesareans. [She had a VBAC.]*
>
> —Lucy T., England

I fear the unknown, and having another cesarean is a "known." Many of the women who schedule elective repeat cesareans list this reason. If you have never had a vaginal birth, if your cesarean went smoothly and presented no complications, and if your recovery wasn't delayed because of a sick baby, infection, depression, or disappointment over breastfeeding problems, then you very well may believe that having a vaginal birth couldn't improve on your previous experience—if you don't have any facts to the contrary, that is.

I worry that I won't be able to stand the pain of a vaginal birth without medication. Labor is painful, often excruciatingly so. But not all labors are equal in their pain intensity.

However, whether your baby is big or little, your labor short or long, you can still plan ahead to reduce some of the pain, even if you ultimately have an epidural. Choose a doctor or midwife who won't make you stay in one position, especially flat on your back. Since hospitals usually require electronic fetal monitors (EFMs) for VBAC labors, find one that offers the kind of EFM that allows you to move around, or consider laboring in a birth center or at home. In addition to your partner, have a woman friend or professional labor assistant with you; her very presence can help to reduce your labor pain (for more about labor assistants, see page 127). Make sure your helpers are aware of a dozen or so non-drug pain-relieving techniques to aid you during labor. Remember that generations of women have made it through the pain of childbirth successfully, even joyously.

Perhaps part of the pain you fear is in the dreaded postpartum uterine exam, in which your doctor puts her hand into the birth canal to check the integrity of your uterine scar just after the baby's birth. According to Bruce Flamm, VBAC researcher, this exam is not very accurate, and the results are meaningless, since a thin scar area requires no treatment. An internal exam could in fact *cause* a rupture of thinned scar tissue, as well as serious infection. Discuss this exam with your doctor in advance, and request that it not be done unless there's a particular reason for you. Usually, the only good reason for this exam is heavy bleeding from an unknown source.

I will get my hopes up, only to have another cesarean and never get over the disappointment. There will always be women who will not have a successful VBAC this time around. Few healthcare providers report a 100 percent VBAC rate. Studies show that your best ally is the belief that you, not someone else, will walk your own path. If you've planned and prepared for a VBAC the best way you know how, and you still have a cesarean, it's because birth is always unpredictable— not because you're defective or you can't stay the course.

> ✐ *A rigid mindset of "vaginal birth = success" and "c-section = failure" does more to contribute to a repeat c-section than to facilitate VBAC. This point needs to be repeated, not just to the potential VBAC mom, but also to those who are VBAC advocates, who can sometimes get a little carried away with crowing VBAC success stories and ignoring those who labored valiantly, gave it everything they had, and still ended up a repeater. Success is in the laboring as well as in the birth.*
>
> —Beth P., California

The triggers associated with my last cesarean will occur again, and I will have another cesarean. Perhaps your last baby was in a posterior or breech position and didn't turn. Perhaps your cervix swelled and labor didn't progress. Or perhaps your last labor failed to progress after you were induced, or you were given an epidural and you stopped dilating. Find out what you can about why your labor stopped when it did. Women's labors have stopped progressing anywhere between 1 and 10 centimeters and even into the pushing stage. Ask the physician or midwife who attended you to check her records. Obtain a copy of your hospital records. Talk with childbirth educators, midwives, and other doctors to get a new perspective. Learn what you can do to avoid the same scenario the next time. Even if the same problems arise, perhaps the outcome can be different.

🖉 *I had always assumed I would try a VBAC, but I still had my doubts. No matter how much I believed cephalopelvic disproportion was the cause of my cesarean, I worried that (1) maybe that wasn't the correct diagnosis; (2) my second baby would be even bigger; (3) each birth and baby is unique; no woman can totally predict the outcome; (4) somehow my cervix just wouldn't dilate past 6 centimeters. What I did know is that my uterus worked just fine in labor and that if I could get past 6 centimeters, I'd have a VBAC. [She did.]*

—Pamela C., Colorado

🖉 *Labor progressed smoothly for a while and then suddenly I heard the dreaded words: "8 centimeters and a thick cervical lip" [the reason for her previous cesarean]. I was offered an epidural, but at 8 centimeters I felt I was too close to cave in to the temptation. Soon, I felt the urge to push. It was overwhelming, but the nurse held me back, saying the lip was still too thick. For two hours I panted through contractions that came one on top of the other. I couldn't have done it without two helpers. My husband held my hand and helped me control the breathing. Leslie, my doula, provided counterpressure on my back the entire time. I could see them tiring along with me. Even so, every time I was checked, there was progress—a point Leslie, Bob, and the nurse strongly emphasized. I reached 9 centimeters and the lip began to thin. Still, the urge to push was almost uncontrollable. Finally, the doctor said, "With the next contraction, start pushing." So I pushed, but not effectively. I needed a moment to make the adjustment, took a deep breath and pushed again. "The baby's crowning," I heard*

Leslie and Bob say. I couldn't believe it. With the next push, the baby's head came out. Leslie told me the head had been born. Both she and Bob later recalled how I looked at her in complete and utter disbelief. And next thing you know, there was John, weighing 8 pounds, 6 ounces.

—Marjolijn B., Virginia

How to Manage Your VBAC Fears

Now that you have read about the most common VBAC fears, you'll need some strategies to help you cope with your own VBAC concerns so that you remain positive and focused on your goal of a successful birth experience.

If you tried for a vaginal birth with your last baby but ended up with a cesarean, appreciate that you did your best. You may find yourself going over all the "what ifs": What if I hadn't had Pitocin (or what if I had)? What if I had waited to have an epidural? Would my body have relaxed if I'd had an epidural sooner? Or that all-time favorite: What if I had breathed better? Join the crowd; you've got lots of company. It's natural for women to ruminate on their birth experiences, whether joyful or disappointing; we need to review them in our minds and in conversations with other women in great detail.

❧ I have been doing VBAC/cesarean prevention work for twenty-five years. All of the women I have been contacted by, or have met as I traveled and spoke, have made the very best decisions that they could make at the time, given who they are, and the information that they had available to them—or the pressure they felt—at the time. It is important to note that "choices" made out of fear are not free choices, and to distinguish between fear and intuition. All of the women and their families were transformed by the outcomes of their decisions, sometimes positively and sometimes not so positively. People should not have to be defensive if things go well, nor should they have to defend the decisions they made if something goes awry. We do our best to predict outcomes, knowing that our powers to do so are limited at best. Birth is a miracle and also a mystery. We cannot necessarily know what will happen when we begin the journey, although we can certainly trust that in most instances, things will go remarkably well.

Accepting that and at the same time eliminating our fear—not our awe and respect—around it, is perhaps one of our most important challenges.
—Nancy Wainer Cohen, co-author of Silent Knife

Get to know women who have had VBACs as well as other people who will support your goal. Although every year more and more women in the United States have VBACs, it's still not the standard. In our Western culture, most women who give birth after a cesarean have another cesarean. It's no surprise, therefore, that most friends, family members, and even healthcare providers have negative programming where VBACs are concerned; it doesn't matter if they know anything about them or not. Try to avoid the worries and concerns of uninformed naysayers.

⬦ *I was so emotionally distraught after my third birth I did not know what to do. I had been disappointed about all my births, but I truly believed in my heart I was going to do it this time, the third time, and when it didn't happen I just did not know how to handle it. I wasn't sure what was wrong with me. All I would do is cry and felt this tremendous amount of guilt. I finally remembered this VBAC group I had heard about and decided to call. The group really knew what I was feeling. They let me cry and let out all of my feelings, where other people kept telling me I should just let it go because I had a healthy baby. I kept going to that group not even knowing if I would have another child. The VBAC group helped me to become more educated about birth than I had ever been before. They showed me I had options and choices in just about every aspect of my labor and birth. So when I got preg-*

⬦ *How to Manage Your VBAC Fears*

• Appreciate that you did your best with your previous birth.
• Get to know women who have had VBACs.
• Understand that it's normal to feel you will fail where other women have succeeded.
• Read and reread VBAC stories.
• Practice visualization and affirmations.

nant for the fourth time, I knew attempting another VBAC was the only way for me, even though everyone other than the doctor, my husband, and the VBAC group was telling me I was crazy for trying it again and hadn't I suffered enough in my three last labors and c-sections. I had my VBAC with a supportive doctor, my husband, and two doulas.

—Dina C., Illinois

Understand that it's normal to feel that you will fail in your VBAC attempt, even though many women have succeeded. The trauma of having an unexpected cesarean, and then perhaps failing once at VBAC, can imprint itself deeply in your mind, leaving you believing that a vaginal birth is just impossible for you. But many women in this situation have succeeded at VBAC. A positive attitude and advance preparation don't guarantee success, but they have made a profound difference for some women who have had VBACs.

❧ It's worth it to try. A big concern is that we know that we can labor and still end up with a cesarean—we've been there, done that. I had two cesareans before I had my VBAC. So why bother going through all that again? Women need to know that there is a physiological benefit to both them and their babies to go into labor; that even if they have another cesarean, most, many women—all the women I've worked with as a doula— don't regret trying. They have a good chance—as good as any other woman—of having a vaginal birth.

—Kathleen F., Ohio

Read and reread VBAC stories, and gain from their strength. Many women who've had VBACs say that reading other women's VBAC stories made a big difference. It kept them going, knowing that women like themselves, or even women who had more cesareans or more pregnancy problems, had given birth vaginally. Some women suggest that viewing birth videos can be helpful as well.

❧ A story has emotional power: it brings meaning, hope, and vision together; it connects body and soul. It can be as simple as a saying or as complex as a biography; it can come from a conversation, a newspaper clipping, a movie, or a myth. A story can bring the power of imagination into a situation. If we identify with the story, it becomes incorporated into us,

and every cell and molecule in our body responds. When a person is in a crisis and uncertain, the right words can be life-sustaining. There is an Aha! response when the soul makes a link between a story and my story, a sense of recognition that something feels intuitively, deeply right; a match between inner inclination and outer configuration. When a patient learns that other patients with this same illness, or the same stage of the illness, recover, it contributes to recovery: if she could or he could do it, then I can, too!

—Jean Shinoda Bolen, Close to the Bone: Life-Threatening Illness and the Search for Meaning
(New York: Scribner Books, 1996)

Practice visualization and affirmations to help your body and your mind know that your past is not necessarily your future. By "visualization" I mean seeing your desired goal in your mind's eye, as if it's already happened; top athletes often use this technique. Different types of visualization have produced good results in many areas of health care. Affirmations are positive statements you repeat every day, especially when you're deeply relaxed, to send your body the messages you want it to have.

Here's a simple way to get into a relaxed state. Sit or lie down in a comfortable position. Close your eyes. Relax your muscles. You can start by letting your shoulders go limp. Breathe slowly and naturally. As you breath out, feel yourself beginning to relax. Feel the tension leave your body. You might want to imagine that you're doing this in a calm and relaxing place—say, at the beach or in the mountains. Don't worry about how well you're doing. Continue this exercise for 10 to 20 minutes. Do this once or twice a day. Your concentration will improve over time, with practice.

While you're in this favorite place, visualize your baby's impending birth exactly as you wish it to be. Be quite specific: think of your VBAC fears and turn them around into positive images and words. (Examples: See your uterine scar getting stronger and stronger. Watch your baby move smoothly through the birth canal. Feel the power of the contractions and know that you can work with them.) Write down your statements and post them around the house or carry them with you in your pocket as daily reminders. Here are some affirmations to get you started:

- I believe in myself and my body.
- My body is always strong and capable.
- I will give birth vaginally with effort, but also with joy.
- I see myself easily getting past where I was stuck in my last labor.
- I enjoy watching my baby start down the birth canal into my waiting arms.

Why Choose a Repeat Cesarean?

Although we often hear of unnecessary cesareans instigated by doctors, and occasionally of court-ordered cesareans, many women in the United States, England, Denmark, Canada, Sweden, Czechoslovakia, Italy, and other nations demand and get repeat cesareans, even when their physicians do not think they're necessary. Worldwide, one in three women who have had a cesarean will not even consider a VBAC with the next baby.

Women's main reasons for choosing an elective (that is, not judged medically necessary) cesarean are to avoid labor pain, for scheduling convenience, for familiarity and security (they'll know what to expect), and fear of uterine rupture. These women don't want to run the risk of experiencing another long and painful labor, only to end up with another cesarean.

Some of the research found that women believed that having a vaginal birth would put them in danger. It's not clear exactly what they meant, because extensive research shows that women experience far fewer problems after a vaginal birth, not the other way around.

Two of the most important ingredients in a woman's decision about VBAC versus repeat cesarean are her knowledge about VBAC and her doctor's attitude. How positively or negatively her physician presents the prospect of a trial of labor determines to a great extent what the mother will want for herself. For instance, does her physician claim neutrality and tell her it's up to her, even though the mother has no information about VBAC? Is she told that the risk of having a baby born with breathing problems requiring neonatal intensive care is higher with a cesarean than the risk of uterine rupture with a vaginal birth? Does she know she can have an epidural to relieve the pain in a vaginal birth? Is she aware that she can schedule an induction, if her reason for wanting a cesarean is based on convenience? Does she decide on a VBAC, only to discover during pregnancy that her doctor wants her to have another cesarean because her baby is "too big" or "not growing fast enough"—diagnoses that are usually questionable?

Women who would rather attempt a VBAC believe a vaginal birth is better for their child. They think having a VBAC is better for their own bodies, too, and they know they'll have a quicker recovery after a vaginal birth. Some want the spiritual, emotional, and physical high of giving birth vaginally, while others have an intense desire to avoid repeat surgery.

Although some doctors refuse women who want repeat unnecessary cesareans, many other doctors believe that they should respect women's preferences, and they are encouraged to do so by the American College of Obstetricians and Gynecologists. Many researchers suspect that an important factor in the support of elective cesareans is the physician's fear of litigation—especially in the United States, but more and more in other countries, too. For example, what if the rare uterine rupture occurs during a VBAC labor that was encouraged by the doctor, and the outcome is the even rarer newborn death? Doctors have indeed lost malpractice suits in cases like these. (For more on malpractice fears, see page 90.)

Although there is physician support for optional cesareans, when that request is reversed—when women express a preference for VBAC—some physicians are not so obliging, and will discourage women from having vaginal births. Truth be told, some physicians just prefer surgery. Doctors can also have higher cesarean rates because they specialize in high-risk cases, which tend to result in more cesareans; however, much of the difference among individual doctors' and hospitals' cesarean rates, which can range from the single digits to more than 50 percent, is choice.

A woman is more likely to have a VBAC when her physician and hospital are committed supporters of VBAC patient education programs. Vermont, for example, is conducting a statewide campaign to educate doctors, hospital staffs, and consumers to decrease the number of elective repeat cesareans. During 1993 and 1994, Vermont's VBAC success rate was 85.7 percent. The Kaiser Permanente Hospital in Riverside, California, kept its cesarean rate to 12.7 percent in 1992, at a time when the U.S. rate was 23.6 percent, by encouraging VBACs. (Repeat cesareans account for about one-third of all cesareans.)

It's not clear who is supposed to decide if a woman has an elective cesarean or attempts a VBAC—the woman herself, her obstetrician, or her insurance company. During the past two decades, women who have private insurance have had a higher cesarean rate than their non-insured sisters, which suggests that it's the money that controls the method of birth. In a 1996 New Jersey study, women with private insurance or HMO membership were nearly seven times more likely to have an elective cesarean as were Medicaid or self-pay patients. Women who are able to pay the thousands of dollars' difference between vaginal and surgical birth will probably always find cooperative doctors. (See "If You Have a Planned Repeat Cesarean," page 167, if you know that a VBAC is not for you.)

If You Have a History of Childhood Sexual Abuse

No one knows the exact figure, but the National Center on Child Abuse and Neglect estimates that one-quarter to one-half of all women have experienced sexual abuse as children—that is, involuntary sexual experience before age eighteen. Some women bury the memory of abuse until it surfaces while they are pregnant or in labor; others have lived with the memories for years.

This history can complicate the decision-making process for women considering a VBAC. Labor and birth use the same organs of the body that may have been involved in sexual abuse. Labor is characterized by deep breathing, sensations of pressure and stretching, sighs, groans, and sometimes screams. Because sexual abuse can have some of the same elements, it's no wonder these memories can flood back during labor.

❧ I had longed for a baby for eight long years. I wanted a baby with every ounce of my being. When I was finally pregnant (after fertility pills, artificial insemination of Larry's sperm—you name it) I was euphoric. I'm sure there were women who wanted a baby as much as I did, but never more than I did. But childbirth had nothing to do with giving birth to a baby. Childbirth had everything to do with incest. I would not allow any family member to even be in the hospital—much less in the waiting area. Except, of course, my husband Larry. He was the only one who "knew"!

—Marilyn Van Derbur, former Miss America, incest survivor, and co-founder of One Voice

According to Penny Simkin, a childbirth educator and expert on the effects of childhood sexual abuse on labor, a woman who experienced abuse as a child may have more difficulty than others with particular aspects of routine maternity care or the labor and birth process. This is because they remind her, consciously or unconsciously, of the trauma she experienced in childhood. She may show some of these characteristics:

1. **Body boundary anxiety,** including worry and sometimes dread of pelvic exams and nakedness in labor.
2. **The need to be in charge,** with inflexible, extremely detailed birth plans and lots and lots of questions for healthcare providers.
3. **Fear of pain or injury to sexual parts** to the point of avoidance of labor altogether by finding ways to not feel that part of her body, either mentally or by having early epidural anesthesia (which deadens all sensation below the waist) or a scheduled cesarean.
4. **Inability and unwillingness to trust authority figures;** or, to the contrary, total meekness, especially if her way of coping with childhood sexual abuse was to be submissive and to imagine that she was invisible.
5. **Resistance to non-intellectual elements of childbirth classes,** such as practicing relaxation exercises while lying on the floor among strangers.

6. **Flashbacks or body memories in labor of the childhood abuse.**
   Some women experience their first memories of childhood
   abuse while in labor in an overwhelming way, filling them with
   fear and sometimes terror.
7. **Shutting down labor altogether when it begins to go beyond her
   control.** (Many women, however, have had their labors stop for
   other reasons, including an epidural or confinement to bed.)

Every woman can see a part of herself in this list if she tries. Many
who have not been sexually abused have had some of these attitudes
and experiences, with the exception of memories of childhood abuse.
The difference is degree. For some women who were sexually abused as
children, the qualities in this list are intense, traumatic, and relentless.

Many women have wonderful birth experiences despite a history
of childhood sexual abuse. But abuse memories can play a role in
some births, and not necessarily a woman's first birth, either. Here are
suggestions that are essential and vital for a woman with this history
who wants a VBAC. However, the underlying themes of building trust
and gaining confidence are good advice for any woman who is pregnant, no matter what her history.

> ❧ *My third birth (after two cesareans) went slowly at first, but with the
> help of an epidural for relaxation and pain relief, I suddenly went from 2
> centimeters to 10 centimeters in no time flat. I have a history of sexual and
> physical abuse from the time I was a small child, and I have a terrible time
> relaxing in labor. This and the fact that my husband slept through the
> whole thing didn't help a lot. I was pretty hurt by the "support" I got from
> those who cared the most. But the birth of my beautiful Brittany was a
> wonderful VBAC.*
>
> *I suddenly found myself pregnant again a short time after she was
> born. As before, I got stuck in labor, so I again took an epidural for the
> pain. I had trouble letting go for what is such a sexual experience. Once
> the epidural kicked in, I was able to relax and let go.*
>
> *—Debby C., Oklahoma*

**Find a VBAC-friendly doctor or midwife who will discuss the sexual
abuse issues that have been provoked by your pregnancy.** Seek out a

healthcare provider with whom you feel comfortable and safe, someone who you feel is your equal, not your superior. This will help prevent feelings of hostility toward your birth attendant that could be triggered by childhood memories of feeling inferior to and helpless with your abuser. If this person is in a group practice, interview the other partners as well. You may find that you're more at ease with a woman, especially one of your own race. Be open and honest. Discuss your abuse history at your first meeting, and ask if she has any experience working with other women with similar histories who want to have VBACs. Ask her what percentage of her patients with a similar history went on to have VBACs, and why she thinks they were successful.

Confirm in advance that this person will have time to spend with you to discuss your worries. Women who have a history of abuse typically need lots of reassurance and advance preparation for the stages of pregnancy and labor. Ask your doctor or midwife how much time you will have with her in each monthly visit; if a typical appointment is 15 minutes from start to finish, it is difficult to have the time you need with that person. Midwives who work at out-of-hospital birth centers or who attend homebirths usually spend more time with pregnant women. Hour-long appointments are common among homebirth midwives in particular.

Discuss your concerns and preferences on a regular basis; that way, when it comes time to discuss your birth choices, there will be no last-minute surprises or disagreements for either you or your birth attendant. Vaginal exams are often a horrible experience for a woman with a sexual abuse history. If you're having a hospital birth, your doctor, although maintaining contact with the nursing staff, probably will not arrive until birth is imminent. That means that a stranger will probably perform the vaginal exams to determine how your labor is progressing. Although research findings discourage frequent vaginal exams, how often you're examined depends mostly on the preferences of individual doctors and nurses. And teaching hospitals, which have interns, residents, and nurses in training, might request more vaginal exams, so that their staffers get more experience. Keep in mind, then, that while there are always surprises in childbirth, you can eliminate some unwanted events by planning ahead and clearing the way for a trusting relationship with your birth attendant.

If having total control is your biggest issue, consider giving birth at home. Home is the only place that is totally familiar, a place where you can be the boss. You must also make certain that is the place where you truly feel the safest. If a homebirth is not the safest prospect for you—it's not for most women—investigate out-of-hospital birth centers, where you will have the next level of autonomy. If a birth center is not possible, analyze birth attendants and hospitals with an eye for their flexibility and willingness to cooperate.

Have someone with you in labor who is close to you. This person should know your history of abuse and be someone you trust—your partner, someone in your family, or perhaps a sister or a best friend. You may also want to have another helper or birth assistant. Find someone who has been with other women in labor with histories like yours. Ask her what techniques seemed to help these women the most.

Find a childbirth instructor who is kind and empathetic. You don't have to make your history public knowledge in order to do this. You'll need someone who will help you learn how to trust your body to labor well, and will teach you to feel confident with surrendering to your body when you are in labor.

Ask doctors or midwives for referrals to therapists who specialize in helping women with a history of sexual abuse. Also get in touch with support groups for pregnant women with similar histories.

> ✎ *I had a background of emotional, physical, and some sexual abuse from my father, and I began having an unsettling feeling that I needed to rid myself of the influence he had over me—he was still very controlling. I also think I somehow knew I was having a girl and needed to change the dynamics of my family in order to protect her. I feel my parents' presence in the hospital waiting room during my first birth was somehow very oppressive, since they demanded progress reports from my husband and would express disgust that I wasn't "doing anything." About six weeks prior to my due date of my second pregnancy, a confrontation arose in which my parents tried to exert undue influence. I took that opportunity to regain my*

self-esteem and regain my life. Although it was upsetting to the whole fam-
ily, I think I was finally free to be the woman I knew I needed to be to
birth my baby.

—*Sunday T., Ohio*

❧ ❧ ❧

If you have a history of childhood sexual abuse, I hope some of your worries have been addressed in this chapter. Now you have more tools to help you understand and work with your fears and anxieties. It's time to find a VBAC-friendly doctor or midwife.

PART TWO

Planning

✐ ✐ ✐

Plan a Successful VBAC

PLANNING YOUR VBAC involves a new way of thinking for many of you. In this chapter, I'll first help you understand why you had your cesarean, and give you suggestions so that you can avoid the same scenario the next time. Next, I'll provide you with tips on avoiding a posterior labor (when the baby is head down, but facing mom's belly instead of her back) or a breech presentation (when the baby is buttocks or feet first), because most of these labors lead to cesareans. Finally, I'll give a new look at birth plans (with ideas on how to make sure they don't become just "wish lists"), along with five recommendations that will help you take charge of your VBAC pregnancy.

Your Cesarean History

Your hospital records will indicate one of the following reasons for your cesarean.

Previous cesarean. This is still the number-one reason for U.S. cesareans, though the number of cesareans for this reason will continue to fall as more VBACs occur.

Dystocia. This is a catch-all label for a too-long labor or a too-large baby for a too-small pelvis. You'll also hear it identified as "failure to progress," often with "cephalopelvic disproportion" (or CPD, when the baby's head is too big for the birth canal) or "posterior labor." Nearly one-third of cesareans are caused by dystocia. Cesareans caused by inductions that didn't work are in this category, including inductions for postdate pregnancies and premature rupture of the membranes.

Fetal distress. As determined by an electronic fetal monitor (EFM), fetal distress accounts for about one in ten cesareans. EFM use continues as a source of cesarean controversy throughout the developed world. In studies comparing the use of the old-fashioned, hand-held fetoscope with the EFM to monitor the baby's heartbeat, the only difference in outcome is that those babies monitored electronically are more likely to be born by cesarean.

Breech birth. This is the cause for one in ten cesareans. A breech position is a buttocks- or feet-first presentation instead of the baby's usual head-first birth position. Three to four percent of babies are breech at birth, and 80 percent of them are born by cesarean. Many breech babies can be safely born vaginally, but a skilled and experienced attendant is essential. Today few doctors are trained to deliver a breech baby vaginally.

Genital herpes, premature birth, multiple births, toxemia or pre-eclampsia, hypertension, and placenta or cord problems. Although these problems occur the least often, they are frequently the most serious. Research has shown that women who are expecting twins can have a VBAC as easily as women expecting one child without added risks, including uterine rupture.

Other Factors That Lead to Cesareans

Your hospital record won't list the other factors that may have led to your cesarean. They include non-medical matters specific to you, your doctor, and your hospital.

Your insurance coverage. U.S. women who have private insurance with a lot of coverage have higher cesarean rates. This is true in some other countries as well.

Your age. The cesarean rate was 24.2 percent in 1994 for women ages 30 to 34, 27.7 percent for women ages 35 to 39, and 31.5 percent for women age 40 and older at a time when the rate for all ages was 22 percent. Although doctors can't be blamed for all the problems that some older pregnant women experience, researchers in a 1990 study could not find a specific physical reason for the higher cesarean rate. They speculated that it was due to "conservative treatment" of older women.

Your educational level. Women with a college degree or higher are more likely to have cesareans.

Your doctor's and hospital's cesarean rates. The cesarean rates of doctors and hospitals vary enormously, even in the same practice or the same city. The higher their rates, the higher your cesarean risk.

Your doctor's cautiousness about malpractice risk. A 1990 report discovered that 44.5 percent of obstetrical claims against physicians involved cesareans, almost always because the doctor didn't do one or didn't do it soon enough. Perhaps your doctor, or one of her partners, faced such a lawsuit, making all of them in the practice especially wary. (For more on malpractice fears, see page 90.)

Perhaps these reasons played a part in your cesarean; perhaps not. One thing's for sure: If you think some of these factors led to your cesarean, you should select your next birth attendant and place of birth carefully to avoid having a repeat cesarean for questionable reasons.

Predicting VBAC Success

Studies show that 70 to 90 percent of women who attempt a VBAC can be successful. Although the beliefs and practices of doctors, midwives, hospitals, and birth centers all play a role in those percentages, another factor for the differences in VBAC rates is why women had their cesareans.

There is no surefire way to predict who will be successful with a VBAC, and there is definitely no precise way to determine who will *not* be successful. In a 1993 study, two-thirds of the women who were predicted to fail gave birth successfully by VBAC. A New York study found that the odds of a successful VBAC increased with the mother's years of formal schooling and were doubled for women who had seventeen or more years of education as compared to those women with twelve years or less.

Statistics show that women who had cesareans for breech birth, those who had a previous vaginal birth, and those who had only one cesarean are more successful with VBACs. However, don't let this deter those of you who have had cesareans but no previous vaginal birth or who have had multiple cesareans.

Some repeat cesareans happen when a woman has a history of herpes. Because the baby can contract herpes as it comes through the birth canal, and possibly suffer from nervous system damage, which sometimes leads to seizures, mental retardation, or developmental disabilities, many women with a history of this disease have had cesareans. However, the protocol has changed in light of further research.

Women who have a history of genital herpes prior to the pregnancy, but who have no new lesions, are now encouraged to have VBACs. Some researchers believe that if a woman gets her first episode of genital herpes during pregnancy, a cesarean is a good idea because there is a 50 percent chance of infecting the baby during vaginal birth. However, according to a 1997 California study, it's very easy to confuse a primary herpes infection with a repeat outbreak if a woman's previous bouts of herpes had no symptoms.

The only way to know for sure if a herpes episode during pregnancy is the first outbreak is to perform careful testing, along with clinical observation, including viral cultures and type-specific serologic testing. To be on the safe side, some physicians prescribe acyclovir (a drug that inhibits reproduction of the herpes virus without killing normal cells) in the last month for pregnant women with no lesions. Adding to this uncertainty is the fact that about 70 to 80 percent of babies who have herpes infections are born to women with no history of genital lesions.

> ❧ *The ninth month came. I took my acyclovir, waddled off to yoga, talked to my doulas when I felt anxious, and had repeated negative herpes cultures. In the fortieth week, Dr. G. examined me, found me fully effaced, and pronounced it "a green light for a VBAC"! My husband and I were thrilled. The story didn't end there. My son was in no hurry to test my body's uncharted territories, and no dilation or other labor signs occurred. I had tried all manner of labor-inducing sure things, and finally told the doctor he could try some gel on my cervix. The second application of gel kicked in with a bang. Within a half hour I was dilated to 4 centimeters. No Pitocin was needed. My beautiful 8-pound son was pushed into the birthing room and our arms about four hours later. Even at the last minute, I panicked and thought the doctors would go conservative and wheel me into surgery. Thank God all turned out just fine! I encourage women to share with one another—especially about herpes, which tends to feel "shameful."*
> —Susan H., Washington

Some repeat cesareans occur with a "too-big" baby. Macrosomia, which is defined as a baby who weighs more than 4,000 grams, or 8 pounds, 13 ounces, is the medical term for a so-called too-big baby. Macrosomia occurs in 10 percent of newborns. Sometimes it can seem that babies are getting bigger every year, but, actually, the average birth weight has increased only two ounces during the past twenty years. When a woman who has a 4,000-gram baby also has a pelvis that is truly too small for the baby, this condition is called cephalopelvic disproportion, or CPD. Unfortunately, the fetal weight cannot be predicted precisely before the birth, either by clinical estimates or by ultrasound. Numerous ultrasound scans are administered every year in an attempt to estimate fetal size, but these scans are often interpreted inaccurately.

❧ *I used the same doctor, and had another ultrasound at the time I was due, when they determined I was carrying a 9-pound, 8-ounce boy. I finally went into labor nine days after my due date. Another ultrasound predicted I would have a 9-pound, 1-ounce boy. My second c-section baby actually weighed in at 7 pounds, 13 ounces.*

—Darla B., Washington

Although fetal size cannot be estimated accurately, moms showed better instincts and guessed the best in one study. When women were in early labor with their second or later postdate pregnancy, their own estimates of the fetal size were closer to the infant's newborn weight than were the physicians' clinical estimates.

Most women who have cesareans for CPD are successful in having VBACs, often with bigger babies. In general, women who have big babies tend to have longer labors, and women who have big babies are likely to have big or bigger babies in future pregnancies. In a 1997 randomized study (considered the gold standard for research), babies fared no better, nor were the cesarean rates any lower, if their mothers' labors were induced instead of letting labor start on its own.

❧ *I had two cesareans for CPD. The x-rays showed an "absolutely contracted pelvis," and my obstetrician told me that "a 5-pound baby couldn't maneuver that pelvis" and asked if I'd had rickets as a child. I am 5 feet 1 inch and wear a size 5 shoe and size 3 dress. I delivered by elective section first a 6-pound, 10-ounce daughter, and later by section a 6-pound, 12-ounce daughter. From there I went on to have a VBAC—my son was 7 pounds. Now I just had another son this past February at home. He was 9 pounds, which is almost double the weight I was told I could deliver.*

—Marianne B., British Columbia, Canada

❧ *My babies weighed: (1) 8 pounds, 13 ounces, (2) 10 pounds, (3) 9 pounds, 5 ounces, and (4) 11 pounds, 12 ounces. Judging by the size of my subsequent babies born vaginally, I'd say the diagnosis of CPD for my first baby [who was born by cesarean] was wrong.*

—Mary H., Kansas

Some repeat cesareans occur with postdate pregnancies. If you had your cesarean because your baby was too big, your chart probably indicated dystocia, because your labor was prolonged. Or perhaps you went past your due date, and your labor was induced, but labor didn't progress, and you had your cesarean. One reason doctors and midwives are concerned about postdate babies is that they are often big babies.

About 5 percent of babies are polite enough to be born on their due dates. Eighty percent of babies are born at term, or between 37 and 42 weeks. Ten percent are born before 37 weeks, and another 10 percent are dubbed "postdate," "prolonged," or "post-term" pregnancies—that is, they go past 42 weeks, or 295 days. Some women have naturally long pregnancies, somewhat in the same way that some women have more days between menstrual periods.

Every year, nearly half a million pregnancies in the United States last more than 42 weeks. Of these, 90 percent result in perfectly healthy babies. The problem is that before birth there is no way of knowing which babies will be among the problematic 10 percent. If you have a 42-week pregnancy, you may want to wait and see; or you may want to discuss other options, such as induction, with your birth attendant. Many doctors are uneasy if a woman goes past 40 weeks, much less 42 weeks. If a prior pregnancy has reached 42 weeks or beyond, make sure you find a doctor or midwife who shares your point of view about handling a postdate pregnancy.

Some repeat cesareans happen because inductions didn't "take." Most inductions do work, whether with prostaglandin gel or Pitocin. But when they don't, it's understandable. It's as if the baby, who is the labor instigator, is saying, "I'm not ready."

❧ *It wasn't until the day after my second son was born vaginally that I discovered that I may have come close to having a cesarean. When my husband saw one of the nurses who had been on duty with me the night before, she expressed great surprise that I had a VBAC. She told him that all the nurses were expecting me to have a cesarean, because I'd had one before, because of my age—I was forty-three—and because the labor was induced. My water broke and my doctor wouldn't let me wait any more*

*than twenty-four hours to go into labor. All of my labor was with Pitocin.
I had my husband with me throughout labor, as well as a friend who had
also been with me at my first son's birth. Both were a tremendous comfort.
What really saved me, though, was a nurse who came on duty at midnight
and offered great encouragement and told me to change positions. As soon
as she helped me, labor changed dramatically. I was at 1 centimeter after
nine or so hours of Pitocin, but then began dilating quickly.*

—Kathryn B., Colorado

The induction that is most likely to end in a cesarean is the one
performed before a woman's cervix is "ripe," that is, softened,
thinned, and prepared for imminent labor. A cesarean is also more
probable after an elective induction for an anticipated big baby. Since
your chances for a VBAC are better if labor starts spontaneously, be
sure to find a healthcare provider who is flexible and who will help
you avoid nonessential labor induction. (For information about medical and non-medical ways to induce labor, see pages 150 and 151.)

How to Recognize a Posterior Position

Posterior labor is one in which the baby is head down, but facing the
mother's belly (see illustration). Babies are in this position 15 to 30
percent of the time when labor begins, and many babies will rotate by
themselves into the ideal anterior (baby's face toward mom's spine)
position (see illustration).

*Facing page: Posterior position of baby
(left); anterior position of baby (right).
The most common position for the baby as he
comes down the birth canal is the anterior
position—head down, facing his mother's
back. This position is ideal, because the
smallest dimension of the baby's head leads
the way through the birth canal. There are
several slightly different anterior positions; the
most common is the one shown here, in which
the baby is turned slightly to the left, known
as left occiput anterior, or LOA.*

*When a baby is in the posterior position,
the baby's head is down, but he faces his*

*mother's abdomen. The baby in this
illustration is turned slightly to his right,
common for babies who are posterior. Most
babies rotate themselves into the ideal anterior
baby's-face-to-mom's-back position. Some
babies, though, are born "sunny-side up,"
with their faces toward their mothers as they
come out of the birth canal. If your baby is
still in a posterior position when labor starts,
sometimes the doctor or midwife can rotate the
baby's head into the ideal anterior position
while reaching into the birth canal during a
contraction.*

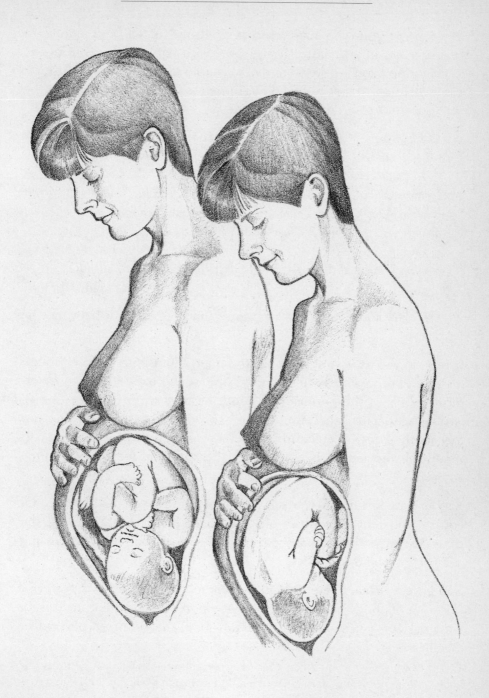

Many of you who had cesareans because of CPD or failure to progress had long, painful back labors with babies who were in the posterior position. Or perhaps you were told that your baby's position was asynclitic—that is, his head was tipped toward one shoulder or the chin was not tucked down on the chest.

> ❧ *I had a c-section with my first baby in 1982 in Columbus, Ohio. The reason given was failure to progress. I labored for many hours, was dilated to 10 centimeters, and pushed for four hours, with no baby. Looking back, I think a skilled doctor or midwife could have turned her head slightly to help the birth. I was in a clinic, being seen by many residents. Later, after another cesarean, this time in England, I was the first woman to have a VBAC after two c-sections at our South Carolina hospital. I had the same problem I had with Baby #1, but the doctor turned her head slightly.*
> —Rebecca B., APO

Here are some signs and symptoms that suggest your baby may be posterior.*

It feels to you as if your baby has too many hands and feet. Although it may be impossible to feel the outline of the baby's back to determine if he's in the posterior position, he may seem to you to be all appendages. This is because the limbs are in the front, and what you feel are the knees, feet, hands, and elbows. When the baby is lying correctly, the movement is all on one side, and you feel half as much activity.

You urinate even more often, and sometimes you leak urine. Of course, you feel like you're already going to the bathroom all the time. The urine leaks may occur because your baby's brow is pressing against your bladder.

You have a urinary tract infection. When your baby is in a posterior position, his body is more likely to press on your bladder, increasing your risk for a urinary tract infection, or UTI. About 10 percent of

---

*The following section is an edited excerpt from "Posterior Labor—A Pain in the Back! Its Prevention and Cure," by Valerie El Halta, first published in 1991. For a copy of her complete article, see the Resource Directory.

> *How to Recognize a Posterior Position*
>
> • It feels as if your baby has too many hands and feet.
> • You urinate even more often than usual, and sometimes you leak urine.
> • You have a urinary tract infection.
> • It may be difficult to hear your baby's heart tones.

pregnant women contract a UTI during pregnancy (many of them also had one or more UTIs before they were pregnant). Symptoms include burning pain during urination, increased frequency of urination, urgent need to urinate but with scant flow, and painful pressure in the lower abdomen or lower back pain. If you have these symptoms, your doctor or midwife needs to test your urine for bacteria. If you have a UTI, it's important to get treatment; untreated UTIs are a risk factor for premature labor. To reduce your chances of getting another UTI during pregnancy, drink plenty of liquids, and remember to visit the bathroom when you feel the urge—don't delay.

It may be difficult to hear your baby's fetal heart tones, or the tones may be indistinct. This is true with either Doppler ultrasound or a fetoscope, a hand-held stethoscope that magnifies the sound of the fetal heartbeat. When this happens, your doctor or midwife will have you roll to the side, and then the heart tones will become more distinct.

A woman who has had a previous posterior labor is much more likely to have another. If you avoid going into labor with another posterior baby, expect a much shorter labor and birth than last time. When your baby is in the "perfect" position—head down, chin tucked in, facing your back—he dilates your cervix much more efficiently as he goes down through the birth canal. As you're looking for a VBAC-friendly doctor or midwife, be sure to discuss your posterior labor history and ask how she can help you if it happens again. (Also read the section in this chapter on turning posterior and breech babies, and the section in Chapter 8 on managing a posterior labor.)

When Your Baby Is in a Breech Position

If your baby is in a breech position—buttocks or feet first—by your thirty-seventh or thirty-eighth week, your doctor or midwife will use a centuries-old procedure known as external cephalic version (often called just "version"). She will place her hands on your abdomen and, with carefully directed pressure and gentle manipulation, attempt to change the baby's position inside the uterus to a head-down position. If a breech position isn't discovered until labor, it's still sometimes possible to turn your baby. While there is no universal list of reasons for avoiding a version, common ones are these: the bag of water has already broken, bleeding is present, or a cesarean is necessary for other reasons. And, in the case of twins, a version should not be attempted before labor and is appropriate only in labor on the *second* twin.

Today a version is usually administered in a hospital. First, an ultrasound scan must determine several things: that the baby is indeed breech, that there is adequate amniotic fluid, that the baby shows no fetal irregularities, and the location of the placenta. No anesthesia is used, but, because versions cannot be attempted during contractions, you may be given a muscle-relaxing drug such as terbutaline, nifedipine, or ritodrine by injection or IV to relax the uterus. Your baby's heartbeat will be monitored during the procedure. In addition, if your blood is RH-negative, and you've not received Rhogam yet in this pregnancy, you will be given it after the version in case there is any fetal-maternal bleeding.

Versions are successful 50 to 65 percent of the time, even if the

Facing page: Footling breech (left); frank breech (right). A baby is in a breech position when his buttocks or his feet enter the birth canal before his head. About 3 to 4 percent of all babies are in the breech position when labor begins. Premature babies are especially likely to be breech, because they're smaller, and some of them haven't settled into a position for birth yet. In a frank breech, a baby has his feet over his head. In a complete breech, the baby sits cross-legged in the uterus. A footling breech—when the baby has extended his foot down the birth canal—can occur only when the cervix is mostly dilated and labor is far along. (Unlike the woman in the illustration, a woman in labor with a footling breech would grimace with great effort.) A baby who is in a transverse lie, which occurs in about 1 in 300 births, is positioned horizontally or sideways in the womb. Nearly all babies who are in a breech position or in a transverse lie are born by cesarean in the United States.

baby's position is not identified until labor. If the version is successful, the baby will usually stay head-down for the rest of the pregnancy. One small study found that all of the women who had previous cesareans and who had babies in the breech position in their next pregnancy had successful versions, with no complications.

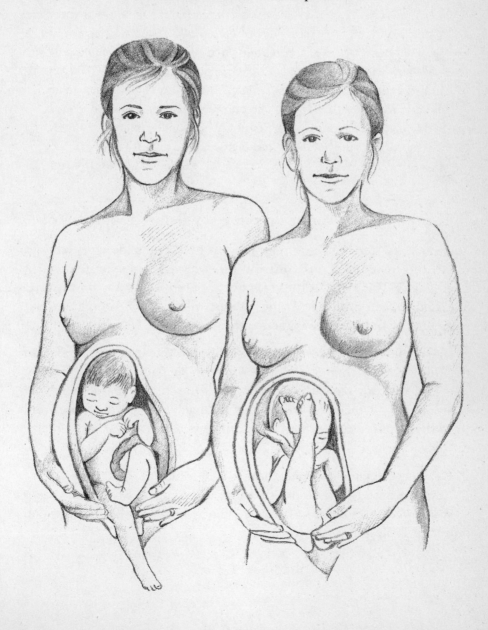

❧ *I made the decision to change ob/gyn practices approximately sixteen weeks into my pregnancy because I saw that my chances of having my physician present during my labor were slim, with five other covering doctors, my history of two previous c-sections, and just a gut feeling that told me to take more control of this birth. To complicate matters during pregnancy, this child was breech and not about to convert naturally to a vertex position. A doctor at my new practice successfully completed a version at about thirty-six weeks, and at thirty-eight weeks my water spontaneously broke. With my midwife's guidance and support, I delivered my second son at a community hospital in Massachusetts. I was very confident going into this delivery. I had thought long and hard and made up my mind what I had to do. I had prepared myself mentally, spiritually, and physically. It was indeed the best thing I had ever done and my greatest challenge.*

—Mary W., Massachusetts

Turning a Posterior or Breech Baby Before Labor Begins

You can take steps during pregnancy to help persuade your baby to move into the correct position, and this will increase your chances of having a VBAC. Some of these suggestions work well for both posterior and breech positions. Some babies will turn after only days, but sometimes a mother must practice these measures for weeks.

1. Do the pelvic rock exercise at least three to five times a day. Get on the floor on your hands and knees with your back straight. Tuck in and pull up your rear, which will serve to arch your back. Hold the position for 10 seconds. Drop your stomach toward the floor, and hold that for 10 seconds. Start over, and repeat ten times. You can also do pelvic rocks, or "tilts," while standing or lying on your side.

2. Get into the knee-chest position for 20 minutes, three times a day. Do this on a bed—the floor is hard on the knees. Keep your knees slightly apart, and bend way over so that your breasts touch the bed and your belly almost does.

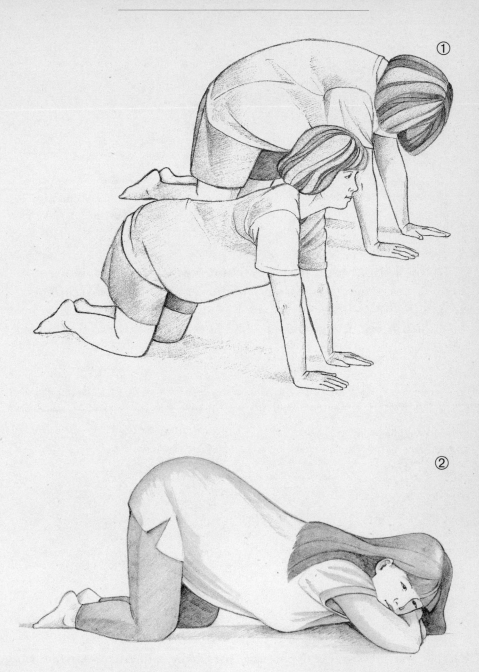

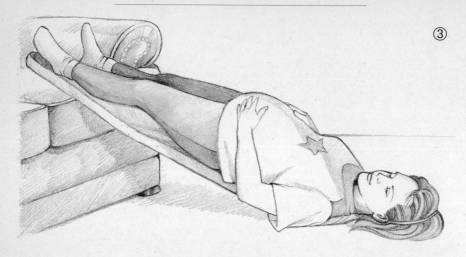

③

3. Lie on a slant board, head down and feet up, for 30 minutes at a time, several times a day. Most women use an ironing board propped against the sofa, with a pillow to cushion the head. You can bend your knees if you like. If you become dizzy, stop and get your feet on the floor.

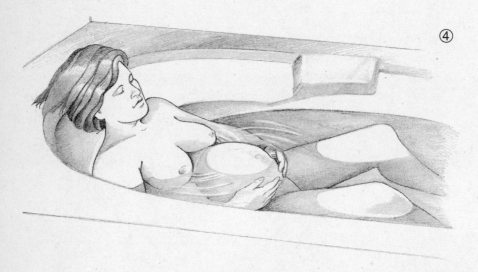

④

4. Take warm baths, gently massage your baby, and encourage him to roll over. Visualize your baby in the correct position. Talk to him; tell him to move into the appropriate position.

🌿 *When I was about six months along, the midwife reported that the baby was in the breech position. This was very bad news, as there are no doctors or midwives in the state of Rhode Island that I am aware of who will perform a breech VBAC. So I read everything I could about turning the baby. I imagined the baby turning, and I placed music near my pubic bone. I tried almost everything that I read about except lying upside down on an ironing board! Meanwhile, I was trying to prepare for the possibility of a second c-section, making it a better experience than the previous one. For whatever reason, the baby finally did turn in the eighth month. [And she had a VBAC.]*

—Wendy O., Rhode Island

A New Look at Birth Plans

The best thing about birth plans is that you have to become knowledgeable about birth to write one. For many women, used to following someone else's lead and doing what they're told, this is a wholly new idea.

Birth plans are written with great promise, but how often do they really deliver on that promise? Perhaps what you want is not routine for the doctor and hospital you've chosen. Sometimes a doctor or a nurse will go out of her way to accommodate you, but you can't count on it. These professionals will do what they think is best. Why should they act otherwise?

🌿 *We got to the birthing room around 1:30 A.M., where my "guardian angel" [the nurse on duty] was waiting for me. I didn't want to fight for the things I needed to give birth. But when I found out that the doctor who had been avidly opposed to my VBAC plans because I had two cesareans was the one on call, I was ready to stand my ground. Then the nurse told me that she had read my birth plan, and she said, "You call the shots." I couldn't believe my ears. And I was elated to discover that I was between 4 and 5 centimeters dilated.*

—Kathleen F., Ohio

Be aware that birth plans often give false hope. You may believe you will get what you want because you have put it in writing, but the signatures of healthcare providers are not legally binding. Many women have discovered that their birth plans are not much more than wish lists. Still, you need to think about your options—writing up a birth plan forces you to organize your preferences. If you don't know your options, you don't have any. These suggestions will help you get what you want for your VBAC.

Think of what each doctor offers as if it were as limited as a fast-food menu. What you can choose is what's on the menu. There's no point in asking for pumpkin pie or chicken and dumplings at a hamburger joint, pizza parlor, or Mexican restaurant, because the restaurant will never have it, not even if you say "pretty please." In the same way, if 75 percent of the women who give birth with the doctor and hospital you're considering have had epidurals, don't say you don't want to be offered any pain medication. Go elsewhere. If all of the patients of the doctor you're considering are hooked up to IVs as soon as they get to the hospital, don't write "No IV" on your birth plan. Find another doctor or midwife who doesn't have this protocol. Many hospitals will plan to have you on an electronic fetal monitor all during labor, because prolonged fetal distress is the early warning sign of the rare uterine rupture. If you want EFM flexibility, find a doctor and hospital that will give it to you; don't just request it on your birth plan. If you want more flexibility in general, don't forget to interview midwives. A midwife offers a "menu" that is almost always longer than a doctor's, especially a midwife who works outside of hospitals.

❧ A New Look at Birth Plans

- Think of what each doctor offers as if it were as limited as a fast-food menu.
- Look for the professionals who offer what you want, instead of trying to fit what you want into what they do.
- Make your birth plan something that works for all of you.
- Be flexible.

❦ I wanted to have a natural homebirth the next time around, but my husband was totally opposed to homebirth. There were no birth centers in our area at the time, so I requested a birthing room at the same hospital where I had had my cesarean. I decided to change to a doctor whose philosophy more closely matched mine, but eventually decided to go to a certified nurse-midwife [CNM] in my fifth month because the doctor wouldn't agree to intermittent fetal monitoring. I found a doula and a direct-entry midwife in addition to the CNM to provide support. I wrote a detailed birth plan and discussed my requests with each member of the birth team. I paid careful attention to nutrition, and exercised throughout my pregnancy, doing aerobic activity, moderate strength training, and special exercises for childbirth. [She had a VBAC.]

—Anonymous

Look for the professionals who offer what you want, instead of trying to fit what you want into what they do. This is true whether you want a high-tech pregnancy and birth or whether you're looking for a midwife to assist you with unmedicated childbirth. As you interview possible doctors and midwives, eliminate the people who you know will not give you what you want. Remember, you're looking for cooperation and enthusiasm, not reluctance.

If some of the healthcare providers you interview tell you that your ideas are unsafe or unnecessary, isn't it better to determine their attitude early while you can still change doctors more easily? When calling hospitals, ask about everything on your birth plan list. Don't assume that if you're breastfeeding, they won't offer your baby formula in the nursery. Don't take for granted that if they have a Jacuzzi for laboring women to help relieve labor pain, it will be available to you. *Ask first.*

❦ I started with a big upscale OB practice with seven OBs and, as I found out, seven different opinions on how to treat a VBAC. One doctor said external monitoring was fine; another wanted an internal pressure catheter, et cetera. At thirty-two weeks, I finally got the nerve to investigate the other OB practices available through our HMO. I actually interviewed the doctors about their VBAC procedures, quite a change from my "trust your doctor" mindset in my first pregnancy. I ended up switching to a *"no-nonsense" HMO group—no fancy examining rooms, no classical music piped into the waiting room. They all knew me as the lady who wants a natural childbirth. But they gave me respect and treated me as an educated adult who wanted to be an active participant in her birth experience. I spoke to all four OBs in the group about my birth plan, brought my doula with me to an appointment with the doctor I was least comfortable with, and took a proactive role in my pregnancy.*

—Alexandra G., Tennessee

Make your birth plan something that works for you, your birth attendant, and your place of birth. List your must-have items on your birth plan in order of importance. Discuss them on a regular basis with your doctor or midwife throughout your pregnancy; this will reduce misunderstandings during labor. Ask your doctor to put the items you've agreed on into the chart that will go to the hospital. If you've done your homework and found the person and place to fit your needs, why would your birth plan need more than a few items?

❧ Yes, there are certain qualities that I look for in pregnant women. I don't know if I can explain it, but basically, does the woman feel that her body is reliable and capable? Is she willing to take responsibility to work with us through the difficult parts of labor? If a woman comes in with a very long birth plan, it seems to spell trouble. Perhaps this is because she doesn't have faith in the process or provider. I look for flexibility and an understanding that in a hospital birth there will be some sacrifices that must be made to hospital routine. What does birth mean to this woman? A great patient is one who is aware of what she wants, why she wants it, is flexible about some things, assertive about the important things, like bonding, and wants no intervention that may sabotage her efforts. She must be somewhat tough about the experience and have faith in her ability to do it.

—Martha Del Giudice, Certified Nurse-Midwife, New York

Be flexible. If you plan to have a hospital birth, as 99 percent of U.S. women do, you may need to deviate from your ideal plan. Birth is too unpredictable to feel convinced in advance that you know how the labor and birth will go, especially in an institution that has its own rules and procedures, independent of your wants and needs.

❧ A problem with a lot of the pregnancy and labor literature, I think, is the emphasis on preparing a birth plan. I felt like I was pretty flexible with my wants, and yet it still didn't turn out the way I hoped for, but I was very satisfied with the outcome. It makes me sad to hear people say they are disappointed that their labor didn't turn out the way they wanted it to. I think saying a woman should make a birth plan gives the impression that we have more control over the process than we do. You just don't know what situations will arise until you are in labor. You cannot make those kinds of decisions before the actual event is taking place. I would advocate education, an open mind, and keeping your heart set on the ultimate goal: a healthy mom and healthy baby.

—Susan W., Washington

❧ I took the VBAC class a bit late, wrote a birth plan, and my husband and I sat down with my old doctor to review it. I thought the doctor quite unsupportive, though my husband's perspective was different. He got along fine with the doctor, laughing and joking while I was trying to discuss matters. The doctor did say that if I didn't dilate a centimeter every hour in the hospital, he would have to give me Pitocin. I suddenly knew if I stayed with this doctor, I would have another c-section. I missed my next appointment, and they never called. Finally, four days before I was due, another doctor agreed to take me, birth plan and all. After two cesareans, this time I had no epidural or c-section.

—Darla B., Washington

Plan a Successful VBAC

Once you understand why you had a cesarean, how those circumstances might affect your next labor, and what you can do to avoid another cesarean, it's time to figure out exactly what you need to do to plan a successful VBAC.

Take responsibility for what happens to you. Many doctors and nurses do not believe they have a responsibility to educate you about VBAC (though it's helpful and appreciated when they do). That's *your* job. You can find information and support from childbirth organizations and teachers, who will have recommended reading lists and

VBAC information pamphlets. The Internet has dozens of VBAC sites, some of which appear in the Resource Directory. When you are searching for your VBAC-friendly doctor or midwife, take into account your cesarean history. If your cesarean was due to a posterior, for example, find a birth attendant who will help you prevent another posterior. Always look for someone, whether midwife or doctor, who has lots of experience with the matters that concern you.

> ❧ *I'd carefully chosen my OB based on his attitude about women's ability to give birth without intervention. I'd chosen the hospital for their "what goes on in your LDRP [labor-delivery-recovery-postpartum] room is between you and your doctor, we have no rules" attitude. I'd chosen my labor assistant because she was able to teach me that there are real ways to make labor endurable, there are real ways to help babies get born, and these ways don't involve drugs or doctors. She would support both me and my husband when we faltered—would keep us true to the path we envisioned for the birth of our baby.*
>
> —Nina M., Illinois

> ❧ *My memory of this period—when my first child was born, in 1986— now is that it was a process of being educated in the ways of doctors and what I as a woman would put up with. I felt lucky to be going to a major teaching hospital, and not a private one where the most restrictive procedures seemed to be practiced. At no time was any philosophy of birth expressed, or were we told ways to avoid unnecessary intervention. I now realize we were incapable of forming any views of our own, [because] in the absence of direct birth experience, I was, between the input of the obstetrician and the physiotherapist, being educated to be a good patient. I'm not trying to be a conspiracy theorist here. I just think that is part of the process of what happens.*
>
> —Anne N., Australia

Have your VBAC at the safest place for you. Research shows that births at birth centers and those at home—when women are in good health and well nourished and have had prenatal care—are as safe as hospital births. A 1989 study of birth centers with certified nurse-midwives showed that women's satisfaction with their births was high and that the cesarean rate was less than 5 percent—one-fifth of the

U.S. rate at the time. Research on the safety of VBACs has used only hospitals, with the exception of one large 1997 VBAC study of out-of-hospital birth centers affiliated with the National Association of Childbearing Centers. Although the information is not available as we go to press, we know that more than forty-five birth centers around the country participated in the study, which looked at more than a thousand VBACs. To date, there have been no published studies on the safety of VBAC births at home.

Healthy babies can be born and good experiences can be had no matter where and how you have your baby. Trust your own opinions. If the risk of uterine rupture is your biggest concern, find an obstetrician and hospital that can perform cesareans in 17 minutes—the optimum time for both baby and mother after a uterine rupture. As you're weighing safety issues and interviewing possible birth attendants and hospitals, ask yourself, "With whom and where would I feel safest?" And when you've made your choice, embrace it as the best option for you.

Acceptance was the most helpful thing in preparing and achieving the VBAC: my own acceptance of whatever labor would bring, and my midwife's acceptance that all would be as it should be. Because I never went into labor with my first, the midwife's absolute certainty that I would this time was reassuring and valuable. Her willingness to be there and to do whatever was necessary was priceless. Another big difference was the role my husband played. Instead of simply being at my side, overwhelmed with the medical atmosphere and essentially helpless and peripheral, he was cook, caretaker, and chief bottlewasher, so to speak. He took care of everyone, and it gave him a concrete and valuable place in the event. We traded fear for love, and it was worth every moment of planning and work involved. I'd do it again without hesitation.

—Juli D., Virginia

Avoid people—whether family, friends, or co-workers—who will discourage you from seeking a VBAC. Protect yourself and your unborn child from criticism of what you know is the right thing to do. Although VBACs are more common than they once were, some people still have negative programming about them, regardless of whether they know anything about them. If you want, give them some reading material on VBACs. If the people closest to you continue to worry and fret, ask them to keep their concerns to themselves while you are pregnant, and have others keep them occupied while you are in labor. Don't feel obliged to keep constantly reassuring the same people that VBACs are safe.

> ✐ *I had a few people—family members—asking if I was sure that this is what I wanted, that is, implying that it might not be the best route to go. My husband felt that it was my body and my decision. We did attend a VBAC class in which the instructor herself had experienced a VBAC and was very supportive. I do recall a couple of times when I felt like waffling on the decision due to fear of the unknown, but the positives, I felt, outweighed the negatives. Do not get frightened by naysayers, and remember it is your decision and yours alone, [because] you are the one whose body and child this affects.*
>
> —Jamie S., British Columbia, Canada

Eat well and exercise regularly. No matter how the babies are born, mothers and their babies always fare better when moms are well nourished during pregnancy, preferably even before conception. The current recommended weight gain is about twenty-five to thirty-five pounds, though there is some evidence that weight gains above that are fine if the mother eats, according to her appetite, primarily foods that build health. Weight gains of less than twenty-five pounds are not recommended. Some women who have had cesareans because they were carrying big babies have been advised to reduce the fat in their diets during the last two months of pregnancy to reduce the risk that the next baby will be even bigger.

Eat fresh vegetables and fruits whenever possible. Pay particular attention to foods that are rich in vitamin E (cold-pressed vegetable oils, legumes, nuts, seeds, whole grains, and dark-green, leafy vegetables). Vitamin E promotes healing and is necessary for tissue repair, and some research suggests it strengthens scars, so stock up (many prenatal vitamins include vitamin E).

Just as a healthy diet benefits you and your baby, so does regular exercise—at least 30 minutes of exercise three times a week. For most pregnant women, the exercise of choice is walking. According to some researchers, other safe activities, even up to an altitude of 6,000 feet, are golf, swimming, jogging, aerobic dancing, cross-country skiing, bicycling, and racket sports.

One 1990 study found that women who continued their prepregnancy running or aerobics programs, as compared to women who had stopped exercising, had fewer cesareans and shorter labors, and their babies had fewer indications of fetal stress. Of course, common sense should rule. If you have any doubts about running or aerobics, discuss it with your doctor or midwife.

> ❧ *On my due date I felt a little different, but I decided to go ahead and go to my noon step aerobics class anyway. On the way home I did start to feel some very mild contractions occasionally. I called the midwife to let her know what was going on. We both agreed that it would probably be hours before I would need her to come to our home to provide support. By 2:15 P.M. I was feeling very mild contractions every 6 or 7 minutes. By 3:30 the contractions were about 3 minutes apart. When my husband got home 15 minutes later, he called the members of our birth team. When the direct-entry midwife arrived, we decided to move to the bedroom for a vaginal exam. On the way, my amniotic sac ruptured. I was at 10 centimeters! I was surprised and glad, and was ready to start pushing. At that point my husband decided to stay at home rather than risk having the baby in the car on the way to the hospital during rush hour. Our VBAC baby was born after about one and a half hours of pushing—four hours after the very first contraction was felt. His Apgar scores were 10/10. I had no tears because of the perineal massage given by my midwife, and after an hour of bonding with the baby, I got up and took a shower.*
>
> *—Anonymous*

Running and aerobics aren't for most women, though. Other research has indicated that regular exercise, including walking, results in shorter labors, especially during the pushing stage. In numerous studies, women who exercise had fewer and less intense pregnancy complaints like morning sickness, lower back pain, headaches, fatigue, and shortness of breath. Many find regular exercise to be a depression reliever as well. Exercise during pregnancy can keep you in better shape after the baby is born, and it can improve your heart and lung capacities.

Squatting is usually not listed as a pregnancy exercise, but it ought to be, because it increases mobility in the pelvic joints. Work it into your daily life—while playing with or helping small children, picking up things from the floor, gardening, or... you fill in the blank. One of the reasons that episiotomies are not common in Asia is that women squat when they go to the bathroom—they don't sit on toilets.

Kegel exercises will strengthen your vagina and birth canal. To do Kegels, first isolate the pubococcygeus (PC) muscle: sit on the toilet, start to urinate, and then stop. That muscle you feel when you start and stop urinating is the PC muscle. Several times a day, make quick squeezes of the PC muscle to the beat of your heart; at other times, hold the squeeze for 10 seconds before releasing. Aim for a total of 15 minutes of Kegels a day. Some women make Kegel exercising part of their lives, pregnant or not. You can do them anytime, anywhere. Practice the "squeeze" at a stoplight or while standing in line at the bank.

Discuss with your healthcare provider what is a reasonable amount of exercise for you, particularly if you have a history of premature labor or vaginal bleeding, or a heart condition, or if she suspects that your baby might be small for its gestational age. Sometimes a regular exercise regimen can mean that your baby might weigh a few ounces less than babies born to more sedentary women.

Always know your options. Understand what's possible. Do your homework about all aspects of a VBAC that are important to you. Speak up and make your preferences known. Change doctors, midwives, or the place of birth if you need to, even at the eleventh hour. Knowing your options will make you much more able to embrace whatever happens. Most of the women who sent in their VBAC stories had either changed doctors or switched to midwives; a dozen changed doctors in the last month of pregnancy. You might think that changing your birth attendant in the last trimester or the last few weeks would be traumatic, but it's not if it's intentional.

It's not difficult to find a doctor or midwife who will take you into her practice at the last minute; just make sure you check your insurance coverage (more on insurance in the next chapter). Lots of people change doctors for all sorts of good reasons. It's important to let the first doctor's office know, but you don't have to be apologetic if you want to change doctors. Once you've selected your new doctor or midwife, either ask for a copy of your file yourself or have your new birth attendant request a file transfer.

❧ *The key was being firm and not being afraid to ask for what I wanted and needed—something very hard for me to do. The whole VBAC experience was incredible. It's so amazing to me that I found I could stand up for myself, my body, and my child and ask for what I wanted from the doctors. It's always been so hard for me to believe that I deserved to be treated with respect by the medical community. I always had looked upon them as "gods" who were in a position of power. It was amazing to me how uncomfortable many of the doctors I interviewed were when I asked tough questions. I realized that the power was inside of me. By taking control of my care, I was able to deal with my fear of the unknown.*

—Alexandra G., Tennessee

❧ *My doctor told me I had a small pelvis and she doubted if I would be able to have over a 6-pound baby vaginally, but that did not make much sense to me. Fortunately, I was going through a training program to become a doula and I learned all about VBACs and cesareans. It was in this program that I found the support needed to have the birth I wanted. So after eight months of prenatal care by the doctor who had delivered Ian by cesarean, I decided to switch to a different doctor, one who had a great track record for successful VBACs and who was very encouraging.*

—Lynelle H., Washington

❧ ❧ ❧

Now that you know at least some of the ways to avoid having another cesarean, it's time to move on to a discussion of medical insurance. An important part of planning a VBAC is understanding your insurance options. When it comes time to choose a VBAC-friendly doctor, midwife, hospital, or birth center, you will want to know exactly what your insurance coverage pays for and what it doesn't, and what you and your insurance company can do ahead of time to line up the people and places you want for your next birth.

CHAPTER 4

𝒁 𝒁 𝒁

Make the Most of Your
Medical Insurance

Become an Expert on Your Insurance Options
What to Do When Your Insurance Company Says No

I N 1 9 9 5 , a hospital vaginal birth averaged $6,378, and a cesarean, $10,678, according to the American College of Obstetricians and Gynecologists. The high price tag for a hospital birth means that, for those of you who have medical insurance, the parameters of your particular insurance policy will most likely determine your choice of doctor, midwife, hospital, or birth center.

Long gone is the dominance of the fee-for-service, or indemnity, insurance plan, which allowed employees to choose a physician and hospital without restriction. Although this option still exists, three out of four insured U.S. workers obtained health coverage through a managed-care plan—usually a PPO (preferred provider organization) or an HMO (health maintenance organization)—in 1995. Under the managed-care arrangement, physicians and hospitals agree to specific discounted prices in exchange for a ready-made list of customers and referrals from others in the plan.

PPOs ordinarily have a much larger pool or network of physicians per plan than do HMOs, and no one physician is designated as the "gatekeeper." Subscribers may change physicians at will as long as their doctors are in the PPO network. If you stay in the network, there is a small copayment. If you go outside of the network, you'll usually be reimbursed 60 to 80 percent, depending on your particular plan.

HMOs usually offer subscribers the least amount of out-of-pocket costs because they feature small copayments, but they also have the most restrictions. HMO plans feature a gatekeeper physician, a family physician that you choose from a list of eligible physicians. Typically, your HMO will require you to consult with this gatekeeper physician every time you want to switch your care to a specialist, such as an obstetrician. (Some HMO plans have loosened this rule, however, so that if you're pregnant you can go directly to an obstetrician.) Giant HMOs, such as Kaiser Permanente, have their own staff physicians and medical offices, and occasionally their own hospitals. If you are a member of an HMO, be sure to go in and get acquainted with your gatekeeper doctor at your earliest opportunity. Take along a copy of your medical history, and bring in any drugs—prescribed or over-the-counter—and vitamins that you are taking.

A cousin to the PPO and HMO plans is the point-of-service plan. This arrangement also features a gatekeeper physician, offering PPO privileges at an HMO cost. Depending on your particular plan, you may be able to bypass the gatekeeper and choose your own doctor for an extra fee.

HMOs, PPOs, point-of-service plans, and even the old-fashioned fee-for-service plans are all bought by an individual company for its employees from one of many giant insurance companies, each of which has accounts with hundreds, if not thousands, of businesses and corporations. Your employer might offer only one insurance plan, but some of you may be able to choose from all of the options outlined here. If your employer offers more than one insurance carrier, you might be able to switch plans only during one designated month in each year.

Unlike the insurance options I've discussed so far, an independent practice association, which is similar to an HMO in benefits, is a group of physicians who contract with several insurance companies—not just one HMO—to offer insurance benefits to you or your company.

A decade ago cesareans added $1.5 billion to the total U.S. tab for childbirth. Today's total cesarean cost is unknown, but surely it's still more than a billion dollars. If your insurance covers all costs for your birth, then perhaps the price of childbirth, whether VBAC or repeat cesarean, is not a pocketbook issue for you. More and more couples, however, are having to make larger copayments for hospital charges, whether for extra days in the hospital or for medications. An epidural costs $500 to $2,500, for example, depending on the hospital and the anesthesiologist. An extra day in the hospital in 1994 averaged $931, up from $245 in 1980. And at least some insurance plans, especially HMOs, encourage VBACs to the point that all cesareans have to be preapproved by the insurance company. If the cesarean is not approved, the doctor does not get reimbursed for the cost difference between a vaginal and cesarean birth.

Become an Expert on Your Insurance Options

Read your insurance booklet to make sure you understand your coverage. Insurance coverage is quite specific; what is covered or not covered varies, as does the deductible, from company to company, plan to plan, and sometimes employee to employee. Don't rely on discussing your insurance options with your co-workers. Instead, call your insurance company (after you've read your insurance booklet) and find out if you have a "wrap" plan, which is often not mentioned in the booklet. A wrap plan provides additional coverage when you are outside the geographic parameters of your policy. Many HMOs have unadvertised wrap plans; if you are nine months pregnant, for example, and you have a wrap plan, if you go into labor when you're out of town your insurance will still cover you. Call and make sure you know which hospitals are covered in your travel area.

If you qualify for Medicaid, check out your many choices. Not so long ago, women who had little income—and, therefore, were eligible for Medicaid funds—had few maternity-care options. Their choices for place of birth were among overworked hospitals and clinics, and a long wait at the doctor's office was a given. But today, according to a 1997 *Wall Street Journal* article, this government-funded healthcare program, which now pays providers more generously than managed-care health plans do, appeals to all hospitals, even those once thought to be only for the insurance-rich middle class. Medicaid helps to pay for one in three births. If you're not sure whether you're eligible, check with your health department. If you are eligible, call local hospitals and ask if they provide Medicaid-funded maternity care.

If you don't have insurance coverage, look into low-cost clinics and hospital programs. Call the local health department and ask about low-cost prenatal programs. Look for hospital programs that feature midwives—they are usually a best buy.

Hospital charges for childbirth vary widely, even in the same city, so call all the hospitals in your area. Some hospitals will deduct as much as 30 percent of a maternity stay package if they're paid in advance; when you're making your calls, ask each hospital if it does this. If you've been directed to the maternity floor and the nurses don't know the answer, ask for the billing department.

If you're comfortable considering an out-of-hospital birth, look for midwives who work at birth centers and at private homes.

Find out how many postpartum hospital days your plan covers. In 1996 President Clinton signed a maternity care bill that guarantees a two-day stay for vaginal births and four days for a cesarean—if your doctor agrees—beginning January 1, 1998. According to this bill, the clock on your hospital stay doesn't start until your baby is born. Prior to this legislation, many plans allowed only one hospital day for a vaginal birth and two for a cesarean. By contrast, in 1970 the average stay after a vaginal birth was 3.9 days and after a cesarean, 7.8 days.

If your insurance doesn't cover a VBAC-friendly doctor or hospital, find out the difference in cost if you decide to go outside your plan. Many plans will partially cover the expense of going to a doctor or hospital outside of their network. Make it easier for them to say yes by documenting your claim. Show them this book and any other VBAC materials you've read. Emphasize that you will save the insurance company at least $4,300 (the current difference in cost between a vaginal birth and a cesarean) if you give birth with a VBAC-friendly doctor and hospital. If you live in a state such as Massachusetts, where cesarean rates by hospital and doctor are published, send a copy of the statistics to your insurance company. Do your homework well in advance, and notify your insurance company *before* you give birth; most plans are more accommodating to out-of-network requests if you make the insurance arrangements before you need the service.

If your employer offers more than one medical insurance option, determine which offerings are more VBAC-friendly. If you are still pregnant when your company's insurance-switching month comes, you have an opportunity to change plans. Examine both plans if you and your partner have separate insurance coverages.

Ask if your plan covers midwives and out-of-hospital birth centers. Sometimes insurance plans offer the hospital services of both doctors and certified nurse-midwives (CNMs). Although information on the average cost for a CNM is unavailable (hospital-based CNMs deliver about 5 percent of U.S. babies), the average cost of an out-of-hospital birth-center delivery with a CNM is $3,600, versus the $6,378 in fees for an obstetrician and hospital. (The birth-center fee is based on those centers that are members of the National Association of Childbearing Centers. Not all birth centers are affiliated with the NACC.) Fees for direct-entry midwives, also known as independent or lay midwives (whose services are not always paid for by insurance companies) range from less than $1,000 up to $3,000. (See Chapter 5 for more details about CNMs and direct-entry midwives; both groups merit high marks for safety and patient satisfaction.)

Find out how to get reimbursed for the costs of childbirth education classes and a birth assistant. Some insurance companies reimburse these expenses, along with those of lactation consultants; but either you, your physician, or a medical facility has to do the paperwork.

Know how much you're willing to pay when the birth professional or birth setting you want is not covered entirely or even partially by your coverage. Some would argue that having this baby is a once-in-a-lifetime experience, one that should be as good and as safe as you can make it.

After your baby is born, check your itemized hospital bill. Numerous overcharges, whether due to computer mishap or carelessness, have shown up on many thousands of hospital bills. Women have been billed for procedures, anesthetics, and other drugs that they never used; one mom even reported she was charged for a circumcision after her daughter was born. If you do not automatically receive an itemized bill because your insurance company pays part of it, call your hospital's billing department and request a copy. Unless you have 100 percent insurance coverage, you may be able to save yourself some money.

What to Do When Your Insurance Company Says No

Despite the fact that many health plans have advisers to help patients with their grievances, only 1 percent of HMO consumers ever file an appeal. Filing an appeal is easy, according to an underwriter at a large insurance company that sells medical plans to hundreds of large and small companies. Patients don't always win, but insurance companies are often accommodating. In disputed cases regarding out-of-network healthcare providers that eventually reached federal regulators, 25 percent were settled in the patient's favor. Surely, many more were settled in the subscriber's favor before they ever left the insurance company. Here are some suggestions:

Be polite but persistent. Insurance companies say this is the key.

Keep notes on every conversation, and write down the name of every health-plan employee with whom you speak. Ask these employees to spell their names, so that your records are as accurate as possible if you need to file an appeal later.

Know specifically why you were turned down. Get a quote for your records. It's okay to tell the person involved the reason for this: you want to be positive of the wording.

Call and ask for the appeals department so you can get your appeal started. Under federal law, HMOs must tell you how to file an appeal. Other kinds of insurance companies are forthcoming as well. Ask exactly what kind of paperwork they need for your appeal.

If you can't get everything you want, ask for a compromise. Maybe you couldn't negotiate total coverage for a physician, midwife, hospital, or birth center that is not covered by your plan, for example. Your insurance company wants to settle with you and close your appeal. Perhaps you'll be satisfied if they reimburse you more than the plan calls for but less than you originally wanted.

If your appeals process gets stuck, consider hiring an independent medical claims adjuster. These professionals are also known as medical claims consultants or medical claims assistants. They speak the language of healthcare company employees and hospital billing staffs. Their fees are often in the $25- to $75-an-hour range, and sometimes several hours' help is all you need. (To find an adjuster, check your yellow pages, or contact the National Association of Claims Assistance Professionals, in Downers Grove, Illinois, listed in the Resource Directory.)

❧ ❧ ❧

Now that you're on your way to being educated about insurance coverage and maternity care options, you can read the next chapter, on finding a VBAC-friendly doctor or midwife—where to look, what to ask, and what research says about your choices.

CHAPTER 5

❡ ❡ ❡

Find a VBAC-Friendly
Doctor or Midwife

Birth Professionals Defined
Finding a VBAC-Friendly Doctor or Nurse-Midwife
Finding a Direct-Entry Midwife
One More Word on Midwives

T HE MOST important factor in determining whether *you* have a VBAC is your choice of doctor or midwife and the place where you give birth. It's not why you had a cesarean, or even how many you had. It's not having a birth plan, or how many books you read. And it's certainly not whether you attended a VBAC class or how many miles you walked during your pregnancy. All of these are significant, but they're not number one.

Midwives help 70 percent of the laboring women in the developed nations of Europe and Asia, according to the World Health Organization. In the United States, however, the situation is very different. According to the National Center for Health Statistics, more than 94 percent of U.S. women who gave birth in 1994 were attended by doctors, whereas only 5.2 percent used midwives. Of those helped by midwives, a mere 40,119 women gave birth at home or in out-of-hospital birth centers.

A note about the studies cited in this chapter: In the research that compares the cesarean and intervention rates of obstetricians, family doctors, and certified nurse-midwives, the women studied were all considered at low risk for complications. If a woman needed a cesarean, she was, of course, referred to an obstetrician; however, the studies attributed the surgery to the midwife or family doctor when calculating cesarean rates.

Birth Professionals Defined

Obstetricians. More women give birth with obstetricians in the United States than with any other kind of birth practitioner. Obstetricians outnumber all the other doctors and midwives who assist women in childbirth, and, as a group, they are far and away the leaders in performing or authorizing labor interventions, from breaking the bag of waters to performing cesareans. An obstetrician is the specialist that a family doctor or a midwife calls when a woman needs a cesarean or has problems beyond the skills of her primary attendant.

One reason that obstetricians have higher intervention and cesarean rates is their "don't-sit-on-your-hands" training. Another reason is the willingness of many to comply with a woman's request for an elective repeat cesarean. The most important reason of all, some say, is the threat of malpractice suits.

Medical malpractice is defined as injurious or unprofessional treatment or blameworthy neglect of a patient by a doctor; what is considered "injurious" or "unprofessional" varies from year to year and place to place. Three out of four obstetricians have been sued at least once, which is many times more than the rate for family physicians or midwives. In 1989 (the latest available data), 44.5 percent of all obstetrical malpractice claims against physicians involved cesareans. Almost all were for either not doing a cesarean or not doing it soon enough. Fewer than 1 percent of malpractice cases in 1989 involved VBAC.

❧ In 1996, a $98.5 million verdict against an obstetrician who performed an emergency cesarean 27 minutes after the first signs of a presenting uterine rupture resulted in the birth of a child with cerebral palsy. As a direct result of this case, at least one medical malpractice insurance company has strongly encouraged its obstetrician members to have every woman contemplating a VBAC sign a special consent form.

One of the statements on this document is "The risk of fetal death or permanent infant brain damage may be as high as 50% in cases of uterine rupture." This consent form vastly overstates VBAC risks and doesn't bother to point out that elective cesarean also has some risks. Doctors generally don't use special consent forms that describe the risks for other obstetrical procedures, even though they may be much more risky than VBAC. For example, cesarean birth of a premature, 25-week fetus has a hundredfold higher risk for neurological problems, as compared to a full-term healthy baby born by VBAC, but there is no special consent form for "Cesarean for Premature Baby."

I believe that the use of this type of consent form will be the finish of VBACs in the United States. A better solution is more caution about VBACs. At my hospital [Kaiser Permanente in Riverside, California], no mother or baby has ever had a devastating outcome as a result of a VBAC, despite a VBAC rate here of nearly one a day. Research reported in 1993 showed that newborns had few problems if surgery was performed within 17 minutes of the first sign of a possible rupture. Our goal should be to improve the response time for emergency cesareans at all hospitals, rather than performing another 100,000 more cesareans each year.

—Bruce Flamm, M.D.*

Family Physicians. Family physicians (also known as family-practice doctors) treat all members of the family, not just women. These doctors not only had a lower cesarean rate (15.4 percent, versus 26.5 percent for obstetricians) in a 1995 Colorado study, but a lower use of forceps, fewer diagnoses of CPD, and fewer low-birth-weight babies. They also had a higher incidence of spontaneous vaginal delivery, VBACs, and vacuum extraction use. Women who gave birth with family physicians in other investigations of low-risk women had lower rates for induction, external and internal fetal monitoring, narcotic analgesia, epidurals, episiotomies, and postpartum oxytocin use. In all of the research on thousands of women, the outcomes for babies born with family physicians were no different than for those babies born with the assistance of obstetricians.

✐ I was the perfect VBAC candidate. My first baby was born vaginally, so I had proven my body could do it, and both babies weighed 7 1/2 pounds. I started writing letters to OBs and family physicians when Lucie was one, before I got pregnant with my third child. This worked very well. As I

*Adapted, with permission, from B.L. Flamm, "Once a Cesarean, Always a Controversy." *Obstetrics and Gynecology* (90) 312–315, 1997.

wasn't yet pregnant, the doctors and I felt no pressure to get things in place right then. After talking to about a dozen OBs and FPs on the phone, I chose a family physician. Molly came early for me, only nine days late. As I was a VBAC, I had to be moved to the delivery room. We'd just gotten into the room when I had another contraction and had to push. Out Molly came, all of her on one push. When Molly was weighed, she was 10 pounds, 1 1/2 ounces.

—Elizabeth H., New York

Certified Nurse-Midwives. The most commonly used midwife in the United States is the certified nurse-midwife, or CNM. A CNM is a registered nurse with two years of advanced training in caring for pregnant women; she usually works under the supervision of a physician. About 90 percent of the five thousand practicing CNMs in the United States work in hospitals and clinics. The remaining CNMs work in out-of-hospital birth centers and, occasionally, at homebirths. (Information about direct-entry midwives who work at homebirths and in some birth centers comes later on in this chapter.) All midwives are trained to help at the estimated 90 percent of births that are free of complications. Like family doctors, CNMs refer to obstetricians those women who need cesareans or who have unique problems beyond a CNM's scope of practice.

A 1997 hospital study that examined all the low-risk births in the state of Washington found that the women seen by CNMs had a cesarean rate of 8.8 percent, compared with 13.6 percent for those who saw obstetricians. (Of course, it's quite possible that women who seek out midwives are more determined to have a vaginal birth.) Other research comparing the cesarean rates of CNMs with doctors shows an even wider spread. In other studies, obstetricians were more likely to use interventions such as electronic fetal monitoring, epidurals, and episiotomies, and were less likely to wait for the placenta to come out on its own after the birth. The CNMs, on the other hand, favored personally supporting women during labor by helping them to change positions and aiding them with breathing techniques. The research findings are always the same: obstetricians use technology routinely and CNMs use it selectively.

When studies compared CNMs to family physicians, there were

fewer differences, although the doctors were more likely to use episiotomies and their patients did have more cesareans. In any of the studies that evaluated mothers' satisfaction with their births, women reported more satisfaction with midwives—either certified nurse-midwives or direct-entry midwives. Part of that satisfaction surely lies in the fact that midwives routinely stay with women in labor, and therefore can be more accommodating. Physicians usually don't come until it's time for the baby to be born.

CNM/OB Practices. CNM/obstetrician practices are common in certain parts of the country, especially in large urban areas, and they come in a variety of combinations. You might see an obstetrician at the first visit, and then rarely after that. Or you might alternate between a physician and a CNM each month. Depending on the number of doctors and midwives in the practice, you might see each individual practitioner only one or two times. Typically, the visits with the CNMs will be longer than those with the doctors. And, as is the case with most group practices, you won't be able to request a particular practitioner for your birth, although you might be able to request that that person be either one of the doctors or one of the certified nurse-midwives. If you choose one of these combined practices, make sure you know in advance which specialist you will see during the pregnancy and whether an OB or a CNM will be with you in labor.

❧ I was going to the same M.D.'s who delivered my second child by c-section, but I was determined to have things my way in their world. Unfortunately, as I continued to see them, it became obvious that a happy delivery with them was impossible. So at thirty-three weeks, I switched to a CNM at a different practice. I had stated that I only wanted a midwife at my birth. The midwives assured me that, if that's what I wanted, that's what I would get. However, they said the doctors had the same philosophy. In the rotation, I finally met Dr. C. We agreed on absolutely nothing. When my contractions began, I learned that it was Dr. C. who would come on at 9:00. We head for the hospital. They began the 20-minute monitor when Dr. C. arrived to check me. At 8:45 A.M., I'm 8 centimeters. Dr. C. says he wants to break my waters. No, no, I told him. "Well, then, you'll labor longer and harder," he answered. I told him that was fine. "Well, then I have

time to move my car," he said nonchalantly, and off he goes. At 9:00, I have the urge to push. One of the nurses checks me, and in a bit of shock turns to the other nurse and says, "She's 10!" There's no lip, just the head—quick, beep him. Shortly after, the head crowned, and right then, with her dad and sisters Kate and Sam watching, Grace Mary was born at 9:15 A.M.

—Margaret K., Massachusetts

Direct-Entry Midwives. Unlike certified nurse-midwives, direct-entry midwives are usually not nurses, and they do not practice their midwifery in hospitals. They enter midwifery directly through independent midwifery schools or through apprenticeship. They pursue continuing education in their field, much like other healthcare professionals. Although CNMs are regulated in all fifty states, not all states have regulations for direct-entry midwives, making the parameters of their legality questionable in those states. It is never illegal, however, for you to give birth at home.

The approximately six thousand direct-entry midwives in the United States attend homebirths or work in out-of-hospital birthing centers. They attend the forty thousand or so women who give birth at out-of-hospital birthing centers and at home each year. (Some midwives believe this number is higher, but even if you double or triple this number, it's still a tiny part of the almost four million U.S. births each year.) About half of these midwives are associated with religious groups; they attend only a few births in any given year, and keep mostly to themselves. Most homebirth midwives are direct-entry, but there are CNMs, and the occasional doctor, who have homebirth practices, too.

Direct-entry midwives refer women to an obstetrician, just as family physicians and CNMs do, if they suspect a problem beyond their expertise. Contrary to certified nurse-midwives, direct-entry midwives are rarely salaried.

Some midwives who attend homebirths have fees on a sliding scale, ensuring that no pregnant woman is turned away just because she can't pay. Others quote flat fees. Many direct-entry midwives work in pairs at a birth. In addition, a midwife will visit you several times in the first days and weeks post partum.

🌿 Non-Hospital VBACs and the Risk for Uterine Rupture

You might be wondering why I've included information about non-hospital VBACs when uterine rupture is possible with any VBAC. The answer is that there will always be reasonable women who choose to have VBACs in out-of-hospital birth centers or at home.

These women believe they have a 99 percent chance of having a successful non-hospital VBAC, and they are correct. Thousands of women have had VBACs in homes and birth centers, sometimes after multiple cesareans, with no problems whatsoever. But when a dreaded rupture happens, the baby's death is likely to follow unless a cesarean is performed within 30 minutes. To avoid any neurological damage to the baby, a 1993 study found, the cesarean should ideally take place in 17 minutes or less.

Sometimes women who give birth at home or in birth centers erroneously believe they can't have a rupture because they are not using Pitocin or prostaglandin gel. Although a rupture is more likely to happen after labor is induced with one of these products, some ruptures have developed without induction. In Arizona, California, and Colorado, and probably elsewhere, babies have died in home births because of uterine ruptures.

Some women who plan non-hospital VBACs choose birth centers that are only a few minutes from hospitals. Others arrange to labor at friends' houses that are quite near hospitals. A few even take nearby motel rooms. While pursuing the benefits of VBAC outside a hospital, these women also take steps to reduce the risks.

Finding a VBAC-Friendly Doctor or Nurse-Midwife

First ask your insurance company—if you are fortunate enough to have medical insurance—whether your plan covers particular doctors, midwives, or out-of-hospital birth centers. Call the maternity floors of local hospitals and ask which doctors or CNMs assist at the most

VBACs. Call the toll-free number 1-888-MIDWIFE to get referrals for certified nurse-midwives from the American College of Nurse-Midwives.

Contact ICAN (International Cesarean Awareness Network) or C/Sec and ask them for local referrals. Call local childbirth educators—both those who teach at hospitals and those who are independent—or call the breastfeeding organization La Leche League (1-800-LA-LECHE) for local referrals. All these groups keep up with the birth news in your area, and usually can tell you who is VBAC-friendly and who is not. Check ads and articles in local parenting publications. See the Resource Directory in the back of this book for addresses of national childbirth education and VBAC organizations.

❧ *It was always my intention to attempt a VBAC. I knew from the beginning that I had to stack the deck in my favor if I was going to have a normal birth. I interviewed all the midwives I could find both in Connecticut and nearby Westchester County, New York. I knew that my best bet would be to have a midwife attending. What I discovered is that there are midwives, and there are midwives. They are not all equal, despite their title. One group of very experienced midwives told me that they would not allow this baby to get as large as my previous child. Well, short of putting me on a regimen of cigarettes and alcohol, I failed to see how that was possible. Another group were very nice, but they practiced in a hospital that required a four-hour separation of mother and baby after birth to observe the infant.*
—Caroline H., Connecticut

❧ *In 1987 I interviewed every doctor I could. I went to the only other OB in this town. He seemed interested in allowing me to "try." I got the distinct impression it was mostly because the other guys wouldn't. He thought it would be OK, as long as labor was during the day only, didn't last too long, the baby wasn't too big, et cetera, et cetera. Even I knew you couldn't control labor that much. I tried the next one on my list, who was about a half-hour away. He was obviously agitated when he saw I had a typewritten list of questions to ask, and insisted on doing a vaginal exam (I should have let that clue me), and he started lecturing me on the dangers of VBAC. The next doc I saw was one recommended by a decent hospital in Toledo as having good VBAC success. He was supportive, but when he found out I'd had a post-op infection, he said it was too risky and would give me a "nice"*

repeat c-section. I continued, and finally saw the guy that was recom-
mended by my VBAC support group friends. He was great! None of his
patients had scheduled repeat cesareans. He had a 95 percent successful
VBAC rate.

—Karen V., Ohio

The questions you ask CNMs who practice in hospitals should be the same as those for obstetricians or family physicians. Address the issues that are most important to you first. You can probably get some of the answers from the person who answers the phone at the office. Ask if there's a fee for a prenatal interview. Most doctors and midwives don't charge, but they do have a time limit. Find out how much time you will have for the interview before you go so that you can pace your questions. This interview will be all talk, and it should not include an exam. After all, you're not going to find out if you're pregnant— you're shopping for a VBAC-friendly practitioner. Take along your partner or a friend to help take notes. Once you have found the right doctor or midwife, you'll continue to have questions each month.

Approximately how many VBACs have you attended? Don't expect a huge number; fifty is a relatively high number, unless the doctor or midwife specializes in them. Out of the 4 million or so U.S. births every year, there are only about 125,000 VBACs. Asking the doctor or midwife if she approves of VBACs will probably not be helpful, but do look for enthusiasm and knowledge. (These qualities are surely lacking if your doctor or midwife asks you to sign the VBAC consent form—a document that exaggerates the possible side effects of a VBAC and that includes none of the risks of a repeat cesarean mentioned on page 19–21.)

In a 1990 American College of Obstetricians and Gynecologists survey, 92 percent of obstetricians said they thought VBACs were a good idea. This was in a year when 22 percent of births following a cesarean were VBAC. Of those 78 percent of women who had repeat cesareans in that year, some wanted the repeat cesarean, and others had physicians who were not encouraging about VBACs. That same ACOG survey found that younger doctors were more interested in VBACs than older doctors, and female obstetricians more than male ones.

Although midwives usually welcome VBACs, not all out-of-hospital birth centers allow them. In general, hospital-based certified nurse-midwives and direct-entry midwives who work in birth centers and in women's homes enthusiastically attend VBACs.

Of those patients in your practice who wanted VBACs, how many were successful? This is just as important as the first question. It's one thing to voice support for VBACs, and quite another to "deliver." Expect a VBAC-friendly doctor or midwife to give you a VBAC success rate of at least 35 percent. (The U.S. average was 35.5 percent in 1995. An "ideal" VBAC rate would be closer to 70 percent, a measure of success often cited in studies.) If that's not what you hear, ask why she thinks her VBAC rate is low. Are her reasons sensible? Or does she have strict rules that can interfere with a VBAC, such as a patient who wants a VBAC must be confined to bed during labor, or a patient must dilate 1 centimeter per hour for a vaginal delivery? (See page 140 for more information on Friedman curves.)

What do you think my chances are of VBAC success, given my childbirth history? Again, look for enthusiasm about VBACs, especially yours. Find someone who treats you as an individual. Most women, regardless of why they had their cesareans or how many cesareans they had, go on to have VBACs if they want them.

 After my daughter was born nine years ago, I had a tubal ligation, think-ing I was finished having children. Well, that wasn't true. My husband and I decided we wanted more children, so I went to an infertility specialist, had in vitro, and I got pregnant with twins. Meanwhile, I became friends with a lady down the street who's a nurse-midwife. She helped me with my fertility shots, and I talked to her about my previous births. She told me that since I was pregnant with twins, they would probably be smaller babies, and there was a good chance I could have a VBAC.

 She induced my labor three weeks before my due date because of my blood pressure and swelling. And the babies seemed to be at a good weight. As soon as I registered at my local hospital and got unpacked, my midwife had me hooked up to Pitocin. I was on it for an hour or so, but nothing was happening, so she inserted two fingers and tried to open the cervix up a lit-

🌿 *Ten Interview Questions for a Doctor or Certified Nurse-Midwife*

1. Approximately how many VBACs have you attended?
2. Of those patients in your practice who wanted VBACs, how many were successful?
3. What do you think my chances are of VBAC success, given my childbirth history?
4. What is your cesarean rate?
5. How do you usually manage a postdate pregnancy or a suspected CPD?
6. What's a reasonable length of time for a VBAC labor if I'm healthy and my baby appears to be healthy?
7. What percentage of your patients do you deliver yourself?
8. How many people can I have with me during the labor and birth?
9. What is your usual recommendation for IVs, Pitocin, prostaglandin gel, amniotomy, epidurals, confinement to bed, EFM (and so on)?
10. How close together are your appointments?

tle. Still nothing happened. As soon as she broke my water, though, contractions began, and that was it.

I delivered the babies four hours later, first a baby boy weighing 5 pounds, 7 ounces, and half an hour later a baby girl weighing 6 pounds, 12 ounces. They have two different birthdays, because he was born 5 minutes before midnight and she was born 32 minutes after midnight. I would do it all over again. I thank God for allowing me to give birth the way I did.
—Chris M., Ohio

🌿 At full dilation the baby went into distress, just like with my first child, Eric. The room went from dark and quiet to light and full of people. The doctor asked me to change my position, and just like with my first birth, I could see the stricken face of my husband and hear the pessimistic voices of the hospital personnel. I also recognized the preparation for surgery that was going on around me. What happened next is as close as I've ever come to a mystical experience. While all this controlled panic was going on, I had this overwhelming feeling that everything would be all right. Claire's heartbeat *stayed between 60 and 100 beats per minute for 20 minutes, but my doctor worked with me. He used suction to help move her while I pushed to alleviate some of the cord pressure. Her heartbeat finally stabilized at safer levels for the remaining 40 minutes of pushing. When she was finally born, perfect in every sense, I was euphoric. Later I had a nurse tell me she had never witnessed such a birth. She told me any other doctor would have wheeled me into surgery. I've often wondered if my doctor just had a feeling everything would be OK. Claire's distress was also cord related. The doctor said her cord, like her brother's, was very long and had gotten wrapped around her neck and shoulder.*

—Lorie L., Colorado

✍ *I had two cesarean births prior to my three VBACs. My first cesarean birth was in 1979. I was diagnosed as having CPD with a baby of 8 pounds, 4 ounces. After twelve hours of labor in the hospital, the baby was a minus 3 station, and a cesarean was performed. The second cesarean was a scheduled one. Although my obstetrician had agreed to work toward a VBAC, and I really wanted to have one, at five days past my due date he felt the baby would be too large. In retrospect, I should have switched doctors at that time, but instead I followed his strong advice to have a scheduled cesarean. The baby was 7 pounds, 13 ounces. This physician commented to me after the birth that there was some malformation of my pelvis, so that a vaginal birth would never be possible, and also referred to a cesarean as a "ladylike" way to give birth.*

—Judy E., Ohio

What is your cesarean rate? Since the care you will receive will be similar to what your doctor does routinely with other pregnant women in her care, beware if her cesarean rate percentage is in the 20s. Ideally, you should find a doctor whose cesarean rate is in the single digits or low teens. In 1995, the U.S. cesarean rate dropped to 20.8 percent from a 1988 high of almost 25 percent. ACOG suggests that a reasonable rate is something less than 16 percent, while other observers believe a reasonable rate is even less than that. Board-certified obstetricians—though essential when you need a cesarean—have the highest cesarean rates with low-risk women. (A physician is board-certified when she has had additional training in a specific field of study beyond

M.D. certification, and has passed a rigorous examination given by a specialty board, such as obstetrics-gynecology.)

To determine the cesarean rates in your area, get a copy of your state's report from Public Citizen's Health Research Group, listed in the Resource Directory.

How do you usually manage a postdate pregnancy or a suspected CPD? The World Health Organization defines a postdate pregnancy as one that lasts forty-two weeks, but some doctors and certified nurse-midwives call it postdate much earlier than that. If your pregnancies routinely last forty-one or forty-two weeks, listen carefully to her answer. Would she automatically schedule a cesarean or induce labor, or would she wait and see, because no research studies report that your baby would have a better outcome by intervening? If your cesarean diagnosis was cephalopelvic disproportion, take into consideration that obstetricians have the highest CPD cesarean rate, family physicians a lower rate, and midwives lowest of all. Obviously, many such diagnoses are wrong. (For more on induction, see page 150.)

> ❧ *I delivered my first two babies with the same doctor. He led me to believe I may have CPD. He definitely felt all my babies would have to be surgically removed. I read about CPD and didn't feel I had any of the risk factors (polio, car accident, small body frame). So before I even got pregnant again, I switched doctors. My new doctor is a woman who has had two cesareans herself. She fully supported my VBAC attempt and my attempt at a drug-free labor and delivery. Next, we decided to switch hospitals. My doctor suggested a specific small hospital. She reminded me that many of the interventions in birth are hospital policy and extremely difficult to avoid. The next morning, my water broke. By the time I called everyone and took a shower, 45 minutes had elapsed and contractions had gone from 5 to 2 minutes apart. Indeed, I had stayed home until transition. I felt I couldn't move. Upon arriving at the hospital, I was fully dilated and ready to push. My doctor held a warm cloth on my bottom, and my doula held a cold cloth on my head. John fed me ice chips. If I wasn't in such pain, I would have enjoyed the service. As the baby crowned, the doctor used perineal massage to get the baby's head instead of performing an episiotomy.*
>
> —Nancy F., Ohio

What's a reasonable length of time for a VBAC labor if I'm healthy and my baby appears to be healthy? Run, don't walk to the nearest exit if a doctor tells you that you are "allowed" to have a VBAC if you dilate 1 centimeter an hour. (A discussion of length of labor appears on page 140.) Ask what the range of time is for typical labors among her patients. Discuss how long she would be willing and comfortable for a VBAC labor to last (ask yourself the same question). Be sure and get the opinion of her partners as well. In a British study that looked at length of labor, researchers discovered greater VBAC success when women had more leeway on the length of labor.

What percentage of your patients do you assist yourself? Many women are surprised when the most VBAC-unfriendly doctor in the practice shows up at their births, but remember: most doctors are in group practices, and that means they take turns being on call for births. Just because your doctor is VBAC-friendly doesn't mean all the partners are. The solution for several women who wrote me was to go in near their dues dates and be induced by the one VBAC-friendly doctor in the practice. If you're unwilling to do that, however, you will take doctor "pot luck" at the birth. So visit all the doctors in the practice before the birth, and discuss your preferences with them. Maybe you'll get lucky and discover that every doctor in the practice is VBAC-friendly. CNMs often work in groups, too.

> ✐ *I knew my doctor would be helpful, since she, too, had a VBAC. However, I went into labor about five weeks early, and my doctor was on vacation. Luckily, the doctor on call asked me how I planned to deliver this time. He tried to stop my labor for twenty-four hours before he decided that it wasn't working. At that point, I had been awake for about forty-eight hours, and I was exhausted. The doctor would not let me give up on VBAC, and I was very pleased with my success. I thought that recovery from my daughter's cesarean birth was fairly easy, but I was amazed at how much easier the recovery was from a vaginal birth. I was pretty much back to normal in a few weeks. I wish I had had more information on VBAC while I was pregnant.*
>
> —Beth I., Maryland

How many people can I have with me during the labor and birth? It's rare for the presence of the partner to be an issue today. However, some doctors and hospitals might have different points of view about the presence of a labor assistant or two. (See Chapter 8 for more about labor assistants.) Because midwives believe in providing social and emotional support to women in labor, they will seldom care how many people you have with you. However, the hospital where they practice may have a different opinion.

What are your usual recommendations about IVs, Pitocin, prosta-glandin gel, amniotomy, epidurals, confinement to bed, EFM, and so on? You will probably get the treatment your doctor or midwife usually prescribes. As I've mentioned, doctors on average use more of these procedures than do midwives, but there are always exceptions. You could also call the maternity floor, and ask the labor-and-delivery nurses what you can expect with a particular doctor or midwife. Some nurses won't discuss this with strangers on the phone, but others will—especially if they are enthusiastic about particular doctors. (For more about routine interventions, see Chapter 8.)

How close together are your appointments? The closer they are, the more you'll wait and the less time you'll have with her. This matters, especially for a woman wanting a VBAC. Many women need reassurance that their VBAC can work, and it's important for the doctor or midwife to take the time to be a supporter every single month.

As you interview, look for someone with "heart." Does she make you feel good about yourself? Does she know your name? Is she familiar with your history? Is she empathetic—can she put herself in your shoes? Her attitude can enhance or inhibit the likelihood of a VBAC. Does she make you feel good about your decision to have a VBAC? Does she listen to you and answer your questions? Does she support you when you voice VBAC fears? Do you feel she's on your side? Will she take your phone calls?

✿ After four cesareans, I went into this fifth pregnancy very determined that this was going to be my way. However, I did have to come to terms with a lot of demons about the first four deliveries, which was tough. During the

early parts of the pregnancy, I was gung-ho and knew I could do this. This was going to be simple. And then, closer to the end, of course, those demons came back to haunt me. The doubts started setting in—"Is this really going to work?" I give my midwife, Linda, credit. She was very patient with me. My visits were wonderful with her because they all were usually over an hour long. She took the time with me to talk to me and listen to me, listen to how I was feeling.

—Jodi B., Indiana

Finding a Direct-Entry Midwife

In many areas, direct-entry midwives are the only practitioners who attend homebirths. To find a direct-entry midwife, contact Midwives Alliance of North America (see the Resource Directory). Or look in your phone book or in a local parenting newspaper for phone numbers of childbirth educators and La Leche League leaders, who can probably provide referrals. You could also call *Mothering* magazine, at 1-800-984-8116; this publication has numerous ads, including some for homebirth midwives and supplies.

Ask your midwife candidates any of the questions listed earlier in this chapter, along with these specific questions, if they apply to you. (Chapter 6 lists questions for midwife-run birth centers.)

How many VBACs have you attended? Look for experience and enthusiasm. Has she worked successfully with women who had the same cesarean history as you? If you had a postdate baby, for example, ask what she recommends for women whose pregnancies go past forty-two weeks (homebirth midwives usually "wait and see"). Ask for references; many midwives will automatically give you the names of the women whose VBACs they have attended. Like many other healthcare professionals, however, homebirth midwives won't treat you any differently just because you have a cesarean history. They believe your labor will be like that of any other woman having a vaginal birth.

How many women in your care have transferred to a hospital? Who is your back-up physician? What back-up hospital do you use? How far is it from my home? How long would it take to drive there at different times of the day or night? If you have no arrangements with a back-up hospital, what options do I have in preparing for an emergency?

The usual reasons for a hospital transfer from a midwife are the mother's request to do so or a labor that is lasting too long. Occasionally a baby is discovered to be breech during labor, which can result in a hospital transfer and a cesarean, especially if it's a footling breech (that is, foot-first instead of head-first). Rarely, a mother needs a very quick transfer for a uterine rupture. If the midwife or back-up doctor calls to say you're coming for this reason, will the hospital be set up for an emergency cesarean when you arrive? (See "Non-Hospital VBACs and the Risk for Uterine Rupture" on page 95.)

If a midwife works with a back-up physician, that doctor will prob-ably meet you at the hospital if you need a transfer. It's encouraging to have a friendly face waiting for you, but this scenario doesn't happen in all states. Several women did tell me about wonderful hospital trans-fer experiences with doctors they had never met before. Occasionally, a homebirth midwife can offer you a combined service: she works with a doctor whom you will see for one or two visits and who will be at the

---

🌿 Ten Interview Questions for Homebirth Midwives

1. How many VBACs have you attended?
2. How many women in your care have transferred to a hospital? Who is your back-up physician?
3. How long have you been a midwife, and how many births have you attended as the primary midwife?
4. What is your training, and where did you get it?
5. What will happen in my monthly visits?
6. Do you attend births when there are twins expected?
7. How do I prepare my house for a homebirth? Can my other children be there with me?
8. How do you monitor labor—do you use a fetoscope or a Doppler?
9. Will you stay with me during my entire labor?
10. What is your fee and what services does it include?

hospital if you need a transfer. If you are concerned about a possible transfer, consider finding a doctor you like and developing a relationship with her even before you conceive. Then, if your midwife says you need a transfer, this doctor can be called in.

> ❧ *Upon arriving, the midwife did a vaginal exam and found I was 8 or 9 centimeters. My blood pressure and temperature were somewhat elevated and my labia were swollen. The midwife decided it would be prudent to transfer to the hospital. I was disappointed, but she assured me I would have a vaginal birth. So into the car we piled, and off to the hospital we went. Labor slowed to a stop for about an hour and a half at the hospital. I must say the doctor and nurse we had were tremendous. They let my midwife and doula attend me with little intervention, and I gave birth a couple of hours after labor resumed. I had my VBAC!*
> —Miriam G., Connecticut

How long have you been a midwife, and how many VBACs have you attended as the primary midwife? It's important to look for experience in a midwife, just as you would with any other kind of healthcare professional. A direct-entry midwife will not give you an answer in the thousands, but, she may well have attended hundreds of births.

What is your training, and where did you get it? Many direct-entry midwives today have attended independent midwifery schools. Some have been educated in European midwifery schools. Several hundred direct-entry midwives have been certified by the North American Registry of Midwives. Ask your candidates if they, too, are certified.

What will happen in my monthly visits? Most visits with a midwife last about an hour, and will take place either in your home or at her office. Prior to the birth your midwife will need to make at least one visit to your home, if she hasn't been there already. Early on in your pregnancy, she will take a complete medical history and give you a physical, including pelvic exam, urine test, blood pressure, and weight check. The last three procedures will be routinely performed at each visit. She may recommend specific prenatal vitamins, and she'll ask that you get blood typing and a complete blood count (or she'll take the blood samples herself) so that she can look for signs of iron deficiency. You will discuss other forms of prenatal testing, and she'll refer you to a physician or lab if you want them. During every visit, she'll ask how you've been feeling, what you've been eating and drinking, what worries and concerns you'd like to share, and how the rest of your family is faring. She'll suggest foods that are especially beneficial to pregnant women and remedies for specific pregnancy-related aches and pains.

Do you attend births when there are twins expected? Some midwives do, but not all. If you're expecting twins and want a homebirth, be sure to find a midwife with lots of experience delivering twins. Ask for references from other women who've had twins at home. A major concern in a multiple birth is prematurity, so if you go into labor many weeks or months in advance, your midwife will transfer you to the care of a doctor.

> ✍ *Our midwife started picking up that second heartbeat and the body parts were all over, so we had a sonogram two weeks before our boys were born. We were still working out an alternative birth plan when the twins decided to come. Born three weeks early and on their father's birthday, Asaph and Noah came into the world as Baby A and Baby B after a quick five-hour labor in the middle of the night.*
>
> —*Trish E., California*

How do I prepare my house for a homebirth? Can my other children be there with me? You can order inexpensive kits that contain all the things you'll need for a homebirth from mail-order catalogs. Your midwife will tell you how to prepare your bed so that it's ready for the birth and your recovery. Whether it's preparing food or keeping track of everyday happenings in a household, there's plenty for everyone to do, including watching the other children. Be sure to line up a cheerful and familiar adult to mind the children as they come and go about the house. If they're awake, siblings are usually nearby when their moms give birth at home. Prepare them for the homebirth by discussing the hard work of labor: how you might look and sound, who will be there to help, what the stages of labor are, and how long the whole process might take. Explain the time frame in their terms—"It will last as long as two trips to the library" or "three 'Sesame Streets,'" for example.

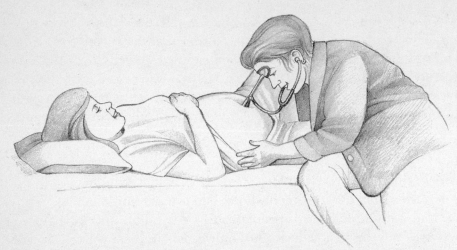

This is the fetoscope, the old-fashioned, hand-held stethoscope that's been largely replaced by the electronic fetal monitor. In the United States, midwives—particularly homebirth midwives—are more likely than any other birth professionals to use this device to listen to the fetal heart tones.

How do you monitor labor? Do you use a fetoscope or a Doppler? Homebirth midwives are more likely than any other birth professional to use the hand-held fetoscope, an instrument that the American College of Obstetricians and Gynecologists says is just as good as an electronic fetal monitor in detecting the fetal heartbeat during labor and for monthly check-ups. Many but not all midwives will use a Doppler—a hand-held fetal stethoscope that uses ultrasound—especially during the pushing stage of childbirth, when, depending on the baby's position, it may be difficult to pick up fetal heart tones with a fetoscope.

Will you stay with me during my entire labor? Homebirth midwives work in pairs; one or both will be with you through most of labor. With long labors, midwives sometimes take turns helping laboring women. As the birth becomes imminent, if they aren't both there already, they will be shortly.

What is your fee and what does it include? Fees for direct-entry midwives range from less than $1,000 up to $3,000. Included in this price are all your prenatal and postpartum visits, along with the birth. Lab tests are usually an extra cost.

Most insurance companies will not pay bills from direct-entry midwives, but they may still reimburse you for your expenses.

In some states, but not all, direct-entry midwives are eligible for payment by the government-funded Medicaid program.

One More Word on Midwives

Unlike doctors, midwives, whether CNM or direct-entry, are not readily available everywhere in the United States. Obstetricians and family physicians who deliver babies outnumber CNMs 11 to 1. In addition, midwives (the word means, literally, "with woman") tend to be a well-kept secret. You may have heard about them, but you may not be quite sure what they do. Maybe you didn't know that midwives, unlike doctors, are trained to stay with you in labor. Perhaps you assumed that the women who go to midwives are uneducated, careless, or part of the counterculture. However, statistics reveal that women who give birth at home or in out-of-hospital birth centers, whether in the United States, Canada, Europe, or Australia, are usually older, married, and white; they are from the educated middle class, are well informed about childbirth, and are very willing to accept responsibility. That's a good description of the women who seek the care of CNMs in hospitals, too.

Many women who choose midwives are familiar with the large body of research that shows the safety of midwifery care for childbearing women who are "low-risk"—a label that covers about 90 percent of pregnant women. (The Source Notes at the back of the book have an extensive list of articles on midwifery and homebirth safety.)

One reason you may not have considered a midwife is that you don't know anyone who has ever worked with one.

On my sister's recommendation, I chose to have a certified nurse-midwife attend the birth of my daughter in 1994 at a wonderful hospital. Although I still thought of midwifery as somewhat radical, I had been told that it was my best bet if I wanted a VBAC. When my midwife explained to me that women attempting a VBAC have a better chance than first-time moms, I knew I had made the right decision. Throughout my pregnancy my midwife asked me questions about what I wanted and asked me to fill out a simple Birth Plan form so that it would be in the file in case anyone else attended my birth. Everything went beautifully. I went into labor at 5 A.M. and my daughter was born at 11:45 A.M. Thanks to the relaxation techniques I had been practicing, it went smoothly and without medical intervention. As a matter of fact, I gave birth to her right into my hands, and I was the one to announce, "It's a girl!!"

—Kathryn L., Illinois

✿ ✿ ✿

There are two crucial pieces to getting a successful VBAC. In this chapter, I've told you about the first: how to find the right VBAC-friendly doctor or midwife for you. The next chapter gives the other piece: how to find the right place for you to give birth.

🌿 🌿 🌿

CHAPTER 6

Find a VBAC-Friendly Hospital or Birth Center

Finding a VBAC-Friendly Hospital
Finding a VBAC-Friendly Birth Center

I T ' S J U S T A S important for you to find a VBAC-friendly hospital or birth center as it is to have a doctor or nurse-midwife who will enthusiastically support your efforts. Some observers say that the place you give birth is the most important childbirth issue of all, because even the most VBAC-friendly physician or CNM cannot be as accommodating as you might want if she is practicing in a hospital that has regulations that make VBAC difficult.

In the United States, 99 percent of births occur in hospitals, including most midwife-attended births. Out-of-hospital birth centers, which started to sprout up in the 1970s and grew more rapidly in the 1980s, are often considered the place midway between having a baby at home and in a hospital. Operated by certified nurse-midwives, direct-entry midwives, and the occasional physician, out-of-hospital birth centers offer low-tech births (only for healthy women) at an affordable cost: an average fee of $3,600, versus the $6,378 for an obstetrician and hospital. The fees at birth centers run by direct-entry midwives might be less.

Some hospitals offer their own birth centers, which are integrated into the maternity wing and are usually staffed by CNMs. Although only 1 percent of births occur outside of hospitals in the United States—a rate that hasn't changed in ten years—the perceived competition from out-of-hospital birth centers and homebirths may have encouraged hospitals to offer more maternity options.

Finding a VBAC-Friendly Hospital

The most important issue to keep in mind when you're searching for a hospital is the enormous differences that exist, even in the same city, regarding options and success rates for VBACs. When you are touring local hospitals and comparing facilities, remember that what is typical care at any hospital is what you will get, too; this is why it's important to match up your preferences with the hospital's routine. The attitude of the nurses about VBAC (you'll get some sense of this when you call with questions and take hospital tours), as well as the time they spend with you, sets the stage as well. If none of the hospitals covered by your insurance plan look VBAC-friendly, call your insurance representative and ask how much it would cost to go to an out-of-network hospital (for more on getting the most out of your insurance company, see Chapter 4).

Some of the questions that follow can be answered by nurses in the maternity unit. For answers to others, call the hospital or nursing administrator's office to find out who can help you. When you're visiting hospitals, ask yourself, In what facility do I feel the safest? That's where it's best to give birth.

🍃 *This is a story of two hospitals located about an hour apart. At Hospital A, within the first two hours I had an enema, shave, five attempts at an IV, several internals—one to show a nurse what 2 centimeters felt like—and then my water was broken. At Hospital B, they've not performed shaves and enemas for the past twenty years. There are no routine IVs; they use external fetal monitors, not internal; and the internal exams were infrequent and very sterile.*

At Hospital A, there is a 95 percent epidural rate—two nurses told me when I had my cesarean that they thought women who didn't get an epidural were crazy. After my c-section, I was drugged so much I didn't wake up for seventeen hours and was not coherent for another twenty-four hours. At Hospital B, the epidural rate is about 45 percent. I was given half of a Tylenol with codeine for hemorrhoidal pain, and ice packs after my VBAC.

At Hospital A, when I breastfed Shane in the ICU I had to go into a back room where there was one low, old, soft vinyl chair. I could have used the rockers in the ICU next to the cradles if I was bottlefeeding. At Hospital B, the nurses actually tucked Megan into my bed for the night and never took her except for a daily weighing. Breastfeeding was encouraged, and they would not give her a bottle or pacifier if I so desired.

— Katie R., Ohio

What is the VBAC rate at your hospital? VBAC rates vary as much among hospitals as do the number of cesareans. Among ten hospitals in north-central Pennsylvania, for example, the VBAC success rate varied from 13.5 to 39.3 percent. An ideal VBAC-friendly hospital will have a 75 to 90 percent VBAC rate, but these percentages are common only in research hospitals with strong VBAC programs. If no such hospital is available, a rate of 35 percent or higher is probably a good target when you're looking for a VBAC-friendly hospital (in 1995, the U.S. VBAC rate was 35.5 percent). Contact ICAN (International Cesarean Awareness Network) or C/Sec (both listed in the Resource Directory) for names of local contacts who will know the VBAC rates for hospitals in your area.

If you have already found a doctor who is VBAC-friendly, but have now discovered that the hospitals where she is on staff are not, an alternative is to find the VBAC-friendly hospitals and then see if they have a doctor or CNM on staff with whom you would want to work.

Which doctors have the highest VBAC rates? An ideal VBAC doctor is one whose success rate is 70 to 90 percent, which matches the rates in research of hospitals that have strong VBAC-education programs. If the hospital staff is reluctant to give you doctors' statistics, perhaps someone will at least give you the names of doctors who attend VBACs there—then you can call their offices directly. Avoid all doctors known to have high cesarean rates, because their VBAC rates will be low.

Do any certified nurse-midwives practice at your hospital? Some CNMs are in combined OB/CNM practices, and others have independent nurse-midwifery practices with physician back-up. If you go to a midwife, you will cut your risk for cesarean by at least 50 percent.

What is the cesarean rate at your hospital? Just as VBAC success rates vary enormously among hospitals, so do cesarean rates. In one area of

---

🌿 *Ten Questions for a Hospital*

1. What is the VBAC rate at your hospital?
2. Which doctors have the highest VBAC rates?
3. Do any certified nurse-midwives practice at your hospital?
4. What is the cesarean rate at your hospital?
5. What is the nurse-patient ratio at your hospital?
6. Are all of your maternity rooms combined labor-delivery-recovery rooms?
7. How many other people can I have with me during my labor and birth?
8. What is your epidural rate?
9. What is your EFM requirement?
10. Do you have Jacuzzis for use during labor?

New York State, for example, the cesarean rate for hospitals ranged from 13 to 40 percent, and in a recent study of all hospitals in the state of Washington, the cesarean rate ranged from 0 to 43 percent (see "Public Citizen" in the Resource Directory for a guide to hospital cesarean rates in your state). Some studies indicate that teaching hospitals have significantly lower cesarean rates overall. The American College of Obstetricians and Gynecologists suggests that a reasonable cesarean rate for obstetricians is something less than 16 percent; maybe that's a good guideline for the cesarean rate of hospitals, too.

What is the nurse-patient ratio at your hospital? Ideally, according to the ACOG, there should be one nurse for every two women in early labor, and one nurse to one woman for active labor and the pushing stage. No one knows what the national average is, but we do know that it's not ideal. The ratio of registered nurses to patients has been decreasing in recent years as RNs are being replaced with less experienced medical personnel. So unless you have a nurse-midwife for your birth, you may end up sharing a nurse for the duration of each shift with at least four, and sometimes eight or more, other laboring women.

A nurse's job is to perform certain procedures for each person under her care, not to make sure that you're comfortable. Since you'll spend most of your labor with nurses—doctors generally don't arrive until the pushing stage—choose a hospital with the most favorable nurse-patient ratio. Make sure you bring your own helpers—your partner and a birth assistant—as well (for more on helpers, see the next chapter).

Are all of your maternity rooms combined labor-delivery-recovery rooms? And if they're not, is one likely to be available should I request it? Most U.S. hospitals now have these rooms exclusively, but in the not-so-distant past a laboring woman having a vaginal birth would have labored in several rooms. First she would be in the labor room, which may or may not have been private. Then, when pushing was imminent, she would move—with great effort—from the bed in the labor room to a movable cart. She would then be pushed down the hall to the delivery room, and would have to move yet again, this time to the delivery table. After the baby was born, she would be taken to her postpartum room.

How many other people can I have with me during my labor and birth? You'll probably want to have your partner with you most of all, but it's important, especially with a VBAC, to consider having a birth assistant with you, too (more on that in the next chapter). Most postpartum floors permit your other children to visit you after the baby is born. However if you want your children with you at some point during the labor, or immediately after the birth, be sure and check with both your doctor or midwife and hospital staff.

What is your epidural rate? Some hospitals have rates of 90 percent or higher; seldom are rates lower than 50 percent. If you know you will want an epidural, that's good news. If you want to avoid anesthesia, however, it's best not to go to a hospital where its use is standard, because that's what the staff is used to offering for pain relief. If a hospital with a high epidural rate is right for you for other reasons, make sure your helpers are familiar with other pain-relieving techniques (see more on epidurals on page 152).

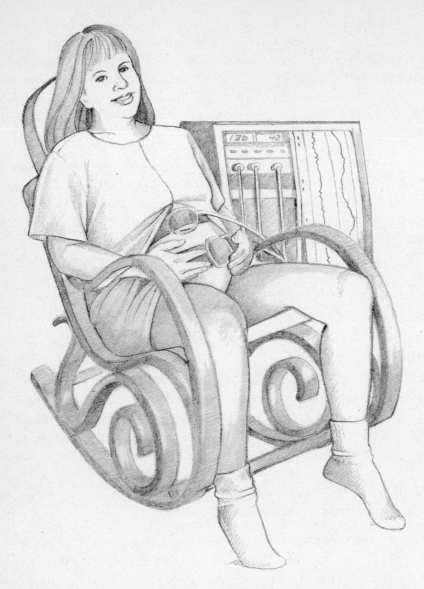

This is the most commonly used EFM device for women in labor. Nearly all women wear the EFM belts while lying in bed. Most hospital rooms have rocking chairs, however, and it's usually possible to sit and to rock while connected to the EFM. This is especially true when you've just entered the hospital and are getting your initial 30 minutes of monitoring. The motion of the rocking can reduce your pain and keep your labor going. Ask about this option when you're looking for a VBAC-friendly hospital.

What is your EFM (electronic fetal monitor) requirement? The EFM device most commonly used in hospitals is one that fits around the mother's abdomen and is held in place by two belts. The mechanism in the lower belt detects the fetal heartbeat, and the one in the upper belt the mother's contractions. (See illustration.) The mother must remain quite stationary while attached to this EFM. A second external EFM device is the telemetry unit, which also utilizes two belts around the mother's abdomen, but allows her to walk around while carrying a small transmitter in her pocket, which radios information to a central monitor at the nurses' station. These two external EFMs use ultrasound waves to do their listening. A third device, the most accurate but most invasive one, is the internal EFM, which measures the fetal heart rate through an electrode inserted into the skin of the baby's scalp, while a catheter placed just inside the mother's uterus measures her contractions. The internal monitor requires that your bag of waters be broken, eliminating it as a cushion for your baby's head. Your baby's scalp is pierced, and there is an increased risk of infection for both you and your baby. Two other monitoring devices are the hand-held Doppler, or Doptone stethoscope, which uses ultrasound to detect the baby's heartbeat, and the fetoscope, which is very much like the common stethoscope.

Virtually all hospitals, doctors, and nurses use EFMs, but every hospital has its own rules about which device to use and how it is used. Nearly all hospitals require a minimum of at least 30 minutes on the EFM, then periodic monitoring after that. They usually require constant EFM use if you have Pitocin or an epidural or indications of fetal distress. And some hospitals require frequent, if not constant, EFM use during VBAC labors, because it is the only way to get an early warning of the rare uterine rupture.

It has always been considered important to monitor the baby's heartbeat during labor. Fetal heartbeats that are too fast or too slow are the markers for fetal asphyxiation—suffocation or choking. About thirty years ago, EFMs began to replace the fetoscope, the old fashioned, hand-held stethoscope used for centuries to listen to fetal heart tones. (See illustration on page 108.) Today fetoscopes are usually used only by midwives, and mostly in out-of-hospital birth centers and at homebirths.

EFMs are excellent devices for monitoring fetal heart tones and for identifying a uterine rupture, but they have been a disappointment in other ways. Researchers early on believed that EFMs would provide crucial information for averting neonatal death, brain or neurologic damage, and cerebral palsy. In the event of a forty-two-week pregnancy, they believed EFMs could warn doctors of impending problems, such as a stillbirth. According to nine international randomized controlled trials—the first of which was published in 1976—EFMs have failed to provide benefits to either mothers or babies over the use of the fetoscope.

In fact, the only change EFMs have brought is a somewhat increased incidence of cesareans. EFMs can produce false calls of fetal distress, resulting in well-intentioned, rapidly performed cesareans. How does this happen? For one thing, EFMs generate vast quantities of data, but, according to the *Cochrane Database of Systematic Reviews*, the largest and most reliable pregnancy and childbirth resource, the interpretation of this data is as much an art as a science. Further, there is no universal agreement on what fetal distress is. Nor is there agreement on what to do about diagnosed fetal distress, or even on what constitutes abnormal labor. Finally, if a woman is strapped to a stationary EFM, she is expected to stay in bed, sometimes without moving around. Staying in one position can slow labor and sometimes cause your baby to have irregular heart tones, suggesting fetal distress.

EFMs are here to stay. Today nurses don't have time to go from room to room listening to fetal heart tones with either the Doppler or a fetoscope. They often care for four to eight laboring women at one time. EFMs produce a read-out regardless of whether a nurse or doctor is in the room. In many hospitals, a duplicate monitor for each woman's EFM is lined up in a row with others in the nurses' station down the hall—a timesaver that allows nurses to pay attention to several monitors at once.

The final reason EFMs are here to stay is because they are so credible in litigation. Although research hasn't embraced EFMs as superior to fetoscopes in monitoring labor, malpractice judges have. In childbirth lawsuits, it's become essential for physicians to be able to provide EFM print-outs in their defense.

Regardless of whether EFMs or another means is used, it is always important for your baby's heart tones to be monitored during labor. The ideal hospital is one in which monitoring takes place in an environment where you can also move around and change positions as much as possible, to keep labor progressing and to reduce pain. Even if you plan to have an epidural, you most likely will not get it until you're dilated 5 centimeters, past the point at which anesthesia can slow or stop labor. (See more on the effect of epidurals on page 153.) The more mobile you are, the quicker you will get to 5 centimeters.

This is why it's important to know the EFM rules at any hospital you're considering. Look first for facilities that use "walking" telemetry EFMs or hand-held Dopplers for periodic checking. Look next for hospitals that do not require EFM use all of the time if you're not using Pitocin or anesthesia. Some hospitals expect you to have electronic monitoring for about 15 minutes per hour, but the rest of the time you are allowed to move around.

Here are some questions to ask as you look for a VBAC-friendly hospital: What is the amount of time I would be required to be attached to an EFM? Do you have "walking" telemetry units? Could a nurse check me with a Doppler periodically at the nurses' station instead of my being strapped to a stationary EFM in bed?

Do you have Jacuzzis for use during labor? Are there enough to go around if several women need them? Since being in water provides relief for so many women during labor, this is not a silly question. Many of the women who wrote to me praised the pain relief of water. Ask if you can have access to a bathtub or shower if the hospital doesn't have Jacuzzis or other tubs containing water jets. If you use a shower, be sure one of your helpers has brought along a bathing suit or extra clothes so that he or she can come in to support you.

Finding a VBAC-Friendly Birth Center

There are at least 150 out-of-hospital birth centers in the United States, most of them accredited by and affiliated with the National

❧ Ten Questions for a Birth Center

1. Do VBACs take place at your birth center?
2. Are you staffed by certified nurse-midwives, direct-entry midwives, or physicians?
3. What is your hospital transfer rate?
4. How many of the women who come to your facility for a VBAC end up with another cesarean?
5. Are VBAC classes, as well as prenatal, childbirth, and postpartum care, included in your fee?
6. How long is a typical prenatal visit?
7. Do you use a fetoscope or a Doppler for prenatal visits and labor?
8. Do you offer pain medications?
9. Who will be with me during labor and birth?
10. How long is a typical postpartum stay at the birth center? Is a home visit part of my postpartum care?

Association of Childbearing Centers. There are also birth centers run by direct-entry midwives that can be located through the Midwives Alliance of North America (see the Resource Directory for addresses). Your cost for a birth-center delivery includes the fee for the midwife or doctor as well as the use of the facility for twenty-four hours or less. Birth centers have no interest in separating you from your baby, partner, or friends. They are not equipped for, nor do they want to give you, a routine IV, or induce labor with Pitocin or prostaglandin gel.

Birth centers are homelike places; some are actually houses where families have formerly lived. A laboring woman has a private bedroom with the kind of bed you probably have in your own home. Some birth centers have extra-wide showers or tubs with whirlpool jets in the private bathrooms. A few birth centers offer water births, meaning that a woman can labor and give birth in the tub. Most birth centers have kitchens available for use, and family members and friends are always welcome.

Do you have VBACs at your birth center? Not all birth centers permit

VBACs, but some do. Ask how many VBACs they have had at the birth center, and what the success rate has been.

Are you staffed by certified nurse-midwives, direct-entry midwives, or physicians? Most birth centers have CNMs on the staff even if doctors are there. If the birth center is staffed only by midwives, ask about their arrangement with their back-up physicians. Some birth centers will ask that you see a physician once or twice during your pregnancy.

What is your hospital transfer rate? Transfer rates vary among birth centers, but a 1989 study showed that about one in six women who planned to give birth at a birth center was transferred to a hospital. The conditions that may require your transfer are: expecting twins or other multiples; a labor before thirty-seven weeks' or after forty-two weeks' gestation; a breech position at full term; the placenta being too close to the cervical opening; and gestational diabetes. Women with a history of high blood pressure, diabetes, cancer, and heart disease usually cannot even enroll at a birth center. Some centers exclude women who take asthma medications. When shopping for a birth center, ask for the names of the hospitals to which women are transferred. How far are the hospitals from the birth center? What is the center's protocol if a woman is suspected of having a uterine rupture? (See "Non-Hospital VBACs and the Risk for Uterine Rupture" on page 95.) Transfer to a hospital does not necessarily mean another cesarean. It makes sense to call the back-up hospitals and ask the questions outlined earlier, although birth center personnel may know many of the answers.

How many of the women who come to your facility for a VBAC end up with another cesarean? Cesareans are not performed at birth centers, of course; women who need them are transferred to hospitals. When asking this question, ask the reasons for the cesareans. The 1989 study cited earlier found that the cesarean rate for birth centers was 4.4 percent at a time when the national cesarean rate was 23.8 percent. Although the National Association of Childbearing Centers is conducting an ongoing VBAC study, and has reports from 42 birth centers on 1,152 births, no results have yet been published. A 1997 California study of 303 low-risk women who had one previous cesarean, however, showed that 98.3 percent of these women had VBACs in a hospital-based birth center staffed by certified nurse-midwives.

Are classes, as well as prenatal, childbirth, and postpartum care, included in your fee? VBAC classes might cost extra, but the rest of the services are usually included. Often the childbirth classes are taught by midwives. The number of prenatal visits is similar to what you would expect from any doctor's office: once a month, with more frequent visits during the last two months. Birth-center staff also typically provide three postpartum visits, with at least one of those in your home.

> ✍ *Tonya and Linda at the birth center were absolutely wonderful. Both of these ladies are direct-entry midwives. They offered a fantastic birth class, which taught us more about preparing for childbirth than any class I'd ever heard of or read about. Pregnancy went very well, with Linda monitoring my weight and keeping me on a low-fat diet to avoid having another 9-pounder to birth. I went to their birth center for prenatals, and all of my blood and lab work was done there. Two weeks before my due date my baby turned breech. But Linda and Tonya immediately had me doing breech tilts in an attempt to have the baby turn before birth. After one week, there was no change, but by one-and-a-half weeks the baby was in position for a normal birth. We praised the Lord and rejoiced that we wouldn't have to do anything further to turn the baby. [She had a VBAC.]*
> — Connie B., the Philippines

How long is a typical prenatal visit? Midwife visits often last an hour. They ask many detailed questions about your habits—what you're eating and drinking, what kind of vitamins you're taking, how much exercise you get, and any issues concerning your family, particular problems, and so on.

Do you use a fetoscope or a Doppler for prenatal visits and labor? Electronic fetal monitors, which were discussed in Chapter 5, are not used at out-of-hospital birth centers. Most midwives use a combination of the fetoscope and the Doppler.

Do you offer pain medications? Some birth centers make pain medication available; others don't. None offers anesthesia such as epidurals. Birth-center midwives use many different techniques to reduce the pain of labor, including helping women to move their bodies into more effective positions or into tubs of water. If only by providing female companionship, midwives make the pain of labor more tolerable.

Who will be with me during labor and birth? Usually at least one of the staff midwives stays with you in labor. Find out what the chances are that a midwife or doctor you don't know will be attending you. Ordinarily, you will have seen all the birth-center midwives during the course of your pregnancy, and there's no limit to the number of your helpers you can bring with you. You will be encouraged not to come in too early, however (as long as everything is normal), until labor is well established, around 5 centimeters dilation. If you do come in earlier than that, the midwives will send you home, or suggest you go for a walk around the neighborhood. .

How long is a typical postpartum stay at the birth center? Is a home visit part of my postpartum care? A typical stay is somewhere between twelve and twenty-four hours after the baby is born. All birth centers arrange for some kind of postpartum home visit. It's unlikely that birth centers will be affected by the U. S. maternity care bill (to be effective in 1998) that guarantees a two-day hospital stay for vaginal births, dependent on a doctor's approval. Birth centers aren't hospitals, after all, and women who give birth there agree with the birth-center personnel in advance on the length of their stay.

❧ ❧ ❧

Perhaps shopping for a hospital or researching out-of-hospital birth centers were new ideas to you. Hopefully, you've done your homework now, and reassessed where you're going to give birth. Even if you've decided on the same hospital you had originally chosen, at least you have made sure that it's the most VBAC-friendly place for you. The next chapter talks about lining up your other enthusiastic supporters: they, too, are critical to your getting your VBAC.

CHAPTER 7

🌿 🌿 🌿

Work with Your Other VBAC Helpers

Your Partner
Your Labor Assistant
Your Childbirth Educator
VBAC Support Groups

IN THE VERY early 1960s in the United States, a woman usually labored alone in a hospital, often with scopolamine (a hallucinogenic drug that caused amnesia so that the woman would not remember her labor) for company, in a bed with sides on it like a baby's crib. A gas mask was usually put over her face for the actual birth, and her husband wasn't allowed in the labor room or the delivery room. He was probably out in the fathers' waiting area, watching a ball game on TV.

ASPO/Lamaze, Bradley classes, and the International Childbirth Education Association were in their infancy, and most women had never heard of them. When I gave birth with no pain medication to my third son, Aren, in 1965, in a large teaching hospital in Kentucky, my husband was the first father ever to be present in a delivery room there. Interns and residents gathered in the hall outside my labor-room door to watch both of us. My, how times have changed.

Nowadays, partners are expected to attend childbirth classes and be there for the duration of labor and birth. Labor assistants (a term I use interchangeably with doulas, birth or labor coaches, birth assistants, or labor support) have contributed the woman's loving touch at numerous births. Childbirth classes have become essential for at least 85 percent of U.S. women. And what would many VBAC-moms-to-be do without support organizations such as ICAN and C/Sec?

Any woman giving birth today benefits from all the help she can get, but especially a woman wanting a VBAC—not because she can't do it, but rather because she needs to surround herself with good information and emotional and physical support from people who believe in her. The importance of supporters to help you get a VBAC cannot be overemphasized.

Your Partner

Your partner's help is like no other's. Although fathers were once excluded from hospital births, today most women find their partner's presence to be the most important one. Your partner's best role is that of the lover offering physical and emotional support, and no one can take that place. Over the years, other duties have been tacked on. Your partner is expected to be a coach and to have the know-how of a labor assistant. (If you have never experienced labor, be sure both you and your partner know what to expect—what you will look like and how you will act and sound, for instance.)

As Jack Hernowitz, a longtime advocate for expectant fathers and author of *When Men Are Pregnant,* has asked, "How can fathers be coaches when they've never played the game?"

❧ *My husband was very supportive of VBAC. Although he didn't understand many of my feelings, he knew that a vaginal birth was important to me. He listened to me read from the many books about childbirth that were scattered in every room of the house. I don't know how many dinner conversations we had about perineal massage, epidurals, and episiotomies, but I'm sure it was more than many men would care for.*

— Chris G., Ontario, Canada

❧ *My husband may not seem to have been very involved with this birth, but right up until my sister had to return home before the birth, he hadn't even planned on being in the same room for the birth. He ended up being right there for me, and though I knew he was terrified, he tried not to show it. I had done all of the reading about birth, and he had never attended any childbirth classes for either child, so I could understand his fear. But he got a crash course and ended up being my hero.*

— Pamela V., Manitoba, Canada

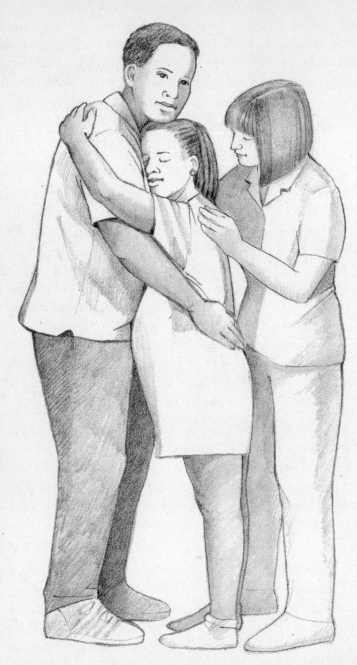

Your partner provides loving support, both physically and emotionally.

❧ *My dear sweet husband squatted behind me and held me up with every push. He talked in my ear and told me how strong I was and how I could do this, how I could birth our baby.*

— *Kristin M., Indiana*

Your Labor Assistant

A labor assistant, or doula, cuts your risk for another cesarean in half—what a boost for a woman having a VBAC! A growing body of research literature reveals that the presence of a female helper reduces requests for epidurals by more than 50 percent, while also reducing the use of oxytocin, analgesia, and forceps. Women who had a labor assistant with them and no epidural reported pain that was no different in intensity than that of laboring women who had epidurals and no labor assistant with them. Best of all perhaps, having a labor assistant at your birth can shorten your labor by 25 percent.

The labor assistant enhances the role of your partner—she doesn't eliminate it—and increases your sense of security because you and your partner are not surrounded by strangers in a strange place. Having other women with laboring women is not a new concept—it's just been newly studied and appreciated. It's a tradition that goes back for millennia and has been practiced in societies the world over. As to why it works, the constant presence of a doula reduces psychological stress during labor, and helps keep the vulnerable laboring woman focused on getting her baby out, rather than on the pain she is experiencing. As necessary as your partner is, there's no evidence that a partner's presence shortens labor or reduces the use of interventions. The woman-to-woman link is essential; it's no accident that nearly all birth assistants have given birth themselves.

Can nurses provide this kind of support? Yes, but nurses come and go from laboring women's rooms, and often care for six to eight patients at once. Nurses don't have the luxury of spending all of their time with one laboring woman. And physicians typically don't arrive until the end of labor (although midwives arrive earlier and usually spend more time with mothers in labor).

❧ I surrounded myself with a wonderful birthing team. My husband's labor coaching and belief in me provided unconditional love and support. A wonderful and tender midwife's commitment and devotion led me through labor with confidence. It was also heartening to share the event with my mother, who witnessed the birth of her newest granddaughter. My sister-in-law, with her love and laughter, added a spark of levity. And there was the proudest member, my three-year-old Raina, whose eyes beamed as she saw her baby sister enter the world.

— *Meryl F., New Jersey*

Certified doulas have more skills than most amateur birth assistants. The two leading training groups are Doulas of North America (DONA) and the Association of Labor Assistants and Childbirth Educators (ALACE). Although the courses that these and other similar organizations offer are not exactly the same, in general they offer workshops of fourteen hours or more over several days. They teach birth assistants how to communicate effectively with families and medical professionals, what to suggest if labor slows, and what techniques might reduce a mother's labor pain. If you want a professional birth assistant, look for a birth coach who has had a VBAC herself, so that when you're in labor you'll have that added confidence in her. Or find a birth assistant who has been with other women who have had VBACs. (See the Resource Directory for a complete listing of organizations that can give you referrals to professional labor assistants.) On average, a professional birth assistant's fee is $300 to $400. Sometimes the cost can be reimbursed by your insurance company (see Chapter 4).

Visalia, California, has a community hospital where 350 to 400 births occur every month. The hospital maternity unit, called the Family Birth Center, provides on-call labor coaches, who have had special training, free of charge to all patients. When asked why the hospital provides this service, lead nurse Christie Caldwell said that staff nurses can't spend as much time with patients as they need to. Other hospitals in California and some in Michigan, Ohio, and North and South Carolina, among other states, have similar programs, and more are in the works. When you're looking for a hospital, ask if it has a labor-coach program.

Is a professional doula always better, however? I don't think so. But there are at least two occasions in which a professional birth assistant is a perfect match: (1) when the appropriate friend or family member isn't nearby, and (2) when neither the only doctor or hospital available to you is VBAC-friendly. In the latter case, a professional birth assistant's extra skills might make the difference between a VBAC and a repeat cesarean.

Over the years, my co-author of *A Good Birth, A Safe Birth,* Roberta M. Scaer, and I have received many birth stories from readers describing the presence of an untrained though often well-read labor assistant who was a friend or a relative. Moms, sisters, and even the occasional teenage daughter have been wonderful helpers to laboring women. Who's to say that the presence of a professional labor assistant would have been better? There are those who believe that in addition to the training and birth knowledge that professional birth assistants have, they have the advantage of not being emotionally involved with the laboring woman or the birth itself. In other words, they can work with a clearer head. But I don't think emotional ties are a bad thing at a birth. Loving ties between friends and family cannot be underestimated. Your mother and sisters and girlfriends are the ones who will be around for your child's birthday parties and other life events, not the birth assistant you hired.

If you are considering having a family member or friend with you, be as careful about choosing that relative or friend as you would be in hiring a certified doula. Don't choose a woman who has had only cesareans or epidurals (if you want an unmedicated birth), who fears

---

🍃 What a Labor Assistant Can Do for You

- She helps you prepare for birth and meets with you several times in advance.
- She nurtures you during early labor.
- She frequently reminds you and your partner of how well you're doing.
- She serves as a buffer with the staff and supports you in having the birth you want.

birth, or who wants to come along just to watch. Look for someone who makes you feel calm, and avoid anyone who might make you feel anxious, or less than able to have a VBAC. If you want to have a trained doula and family member all rolled up into one, ask your friend or relative to take the labor-assistant training. Some women think it's best to have both a friend or relative *and* a professional birth assistant at hand during labor.

Whether you have one birth assistant or two or more, here are some ways they can help you:

A labor assistant helps you prepare for birth and meets with you several times in advance. Some pregnant women find a birth assistant long before they check into birth classes; others sign up for classes first. It's important to meet with your birth assistant several times before the labor so that you feel you can trust this person and have confidence in her ability to help you. If you are hiring a certified doula, ask for references from other clients.

Professional or amateur, a birth assistant needs to know what you want from her. Will you want her to offer a variety of pain-relieving techniques? Will you want her to discuss certain issues with the hospital staff? When you speak to the hospital and doctor, for instance, you both agree that you need to use the electronic fetal monitor for only the first 30 minutes after you have checked in. You remember that the last time you gave birth, however, you were given the same promise, to no avail. There wasn't anyone around to disconnect you from the monitor when the 30 minutes were up. This time, if the same thing happens, you want your birth assistant either to disconnect the monitor herself or to go find a staff member who will.

❧ *When I reached the second trimester and we were informed that we would very likely have a successful pregnancy, we began our search for a doula. I knew I wanted a woman on my birthing team. The woman we chose was our childbirth class teacher who also gave a special class on VBACs which we attended. Our doula reported that with the low and horizontal incision, the danger of rupture is almost nonexistent. I was reassured. And, frankly, she didn't believe I had a small pelvis either, but she said if I was worried, there were visualizations and physical exercises that*

*literally widen the region. She taught them to me and my husband and we
went to work. My doula was instrumental in helping me to build a strong
belief in myself. At age 41, seven miscarriages later, and after sixteen hours
of labor, assisted by my OB, a doula, my husband, and many friends and
family, I gave birth to our son.*

— Michelle H., Oregon

**A labor assistant nurtures you during early labor, whether at home or
in the hospital.** She may rub your back and massage your legs. She'll
know many pain-relieving techniques, from getting into water with her
help to changing positions with her support. (If your doula is a friend
or family member, give her books to read that describe her duties. Ask
your childbirth educator for suggestions.) Some birth assistants are
also midwives or nurses, and as such are trained to examine you and
tell you how much you are dilated while you are still at home.

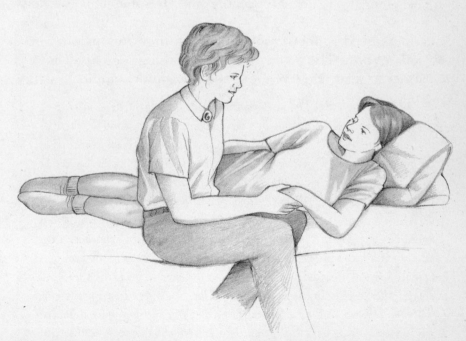

*Your labor assistant provides nurturing encouragement and also communicates with hospital
staff to help you have the birth experience you want.*

❧ *Having had an emergency cesarean with my first child, I was quite nervous about delivering my second child. Bonny, our doula, explained how together as a team we could handle the pain of the contractions and how using different positions would enable an easier delivery. Again, I had a repeat of back labor, but this time, I wasn't lying flat on my back with a monitor on my stomach. Instead, I was up walking around the hallways and using the handrails as a squatting bar with my husband and my doula taking turns massaging my lower back. When I would say, "I can't do this anymore," it was my doula who was right there with the right things to say. She was extremely positive and gave me the support I needed to continue.*

— *Bunny P., New Jersey*

A labor assistant frequently reminds you and your partner of how well you're doing. Laboring women *never* benefit from negative comments, no matter how well meaning. Many women have been told some variation of the following by hospital staff: "Your labor is so slow." "If you don't get going, we're going to section you." "It is shameful how noisy you are."

Partners need support, too. Sometimes they are anxious, especially with a VBAC. The doula provides a soothing presence, allowing the partner to relax and lavish love and care on the mother.

❧ *Leslie's water broke late in the evening and her contractions were coming extremely hard. Leslie was by now completely out of control. She was thrashing under the force of the contractions. Our doula, Debbie, met us at the birthing room and immediately stepped in and began to calm Leslie. She was able to relax Leslie and slow down the rapid-fire contractions. Memories of our first birthing experience came flooding down upon both of us. I left the room to speak to our doctor. I returned to the room and I was immediately signaled to by our doula with a wave of her hand across her face to remain completely silent. What took place in front of my eyes was nothing short of a miracle. Our doula placed her hand on Leslie's forehead and told her to visualize a perfectly calm lake. She asked Leslie to imagine a pebble dropped in the water and to become one of the ripples that was moving away from where the pebble had entered the water. After the visualization technique started to take effect, a great calm came over Leslie. It was as if Debbie had waved a magic wand over the head of Leslie. The contractions began to be spaced from every 20 seconds to over a minute apart. The contractions were farther apart and more powerful and more effective. We were on our way. We moved into the transition phase without any drugs.*

— Jay E. and Leslie H., Illinois

The labor assistant serves as a buffer with the staff and supports you in having the birth you want. She'll remind the staff that you want to walk during labor, and she'll make it possible by dragging along your IV pole. She'll inform the nursery staff that you don't want your baby to be given formula because you're breastfeeding. A good labor assistant is nonjudgmental about your labor choices, whether you want an epidural or a drug-free birth. She's on your side, and she'll be there to help and comfort you no matter what decisions you make.

Your Childbirth Educator

If you had good childbirth classes during your prior pregnancy, you probably don't need to repeat those lessons. Even if you didn't take classes, you know all about cesareans, baby care, and postpartum adjustments.

With this pregnancy, it's more appropriate to discuss your VBAC fears and specific steps to take during labor to avoid another cesarean. It's time for a VBAC class—often just a one-time or weekend meeting instead of the usual six-week course, taught in a group setting or just for you and your partner. You can have a VBAC without taking a class, but most women find VBAC classes very valuable. The ideal teacher is one who has had a VBAC herself.

❧ Mother-Helpers

Having help when you get home is always a good plan. If friends and family members aren't available, you might hire a mother-helper or postpartum doula (see the Resource Directory). She will come in and do whatever household duties you need: cleaning, laundry, cooking, or watching your other children. Many mother-helpers are trained breastfeeding helpers as well, and may even be covered by your insurance policy.

❧ *All my classes are private with only one couple. I tailor my class to their needs. If this includes a VBAC, then we talk more about how their last birth went, how they felt, what they want different this time, and how to maximize their chances of a VBAC. In this respect, I guess it is different than when I teach a first-timer class. If I am doing labor support for them also, I spend a lot of time on the phone with them prior to labor answering more questions and supporting them when they worry. Many of the women I work with—and I must admit, I myself worried a lot over my own VBACs—are really concerned that they can do it. Focusing on birth stories is so much better than quoting statistics. Numbers mean nothing when it is you facing the challenge. Many of my clients have chosen me because I have had VBACs—living proof that it can be done.*

— Toni R., Oregon

❧ *The in-hospital VBAC class was taught by a nurse who had herself had a VBAC. She discussed with each of us what our particular stumbling block had been in labor. Then she gave us each an assignment. Mine was to go home, find an object 10 centimeters in diameter and trace it over and over, and put the drawings all over the house, the car, wherever I would see them most. She was also the first childbirth instructor to mention the word "pain" to me. She asked us how were we prepared to handle the pain of labor this time around. She wasn't shrouding the very real pain of labor in terms like "discomfort" like my previous instructor had.*

— Caroline H., Connecticut

Some childbirth teachers are independent, whereas others teach hospital-sponsored classes. Instructors are often affiliated with either ALACE, ASPO/Lamaze, Birth Works, Bradley, or ICEA (all of which are listed in the Resource Directory). ALACE, Birth Works, and Bradley are thought to be more consumer oriented, with an emphasis on learning about your options. When you call around to find the VBAC class for you, however, the key is to ask teachers how many VBAC couples they have taught and how many actually went on to have VBACs.

❧ *Early on in my eighth pregnancy after seven cesareans, I began having thoughts and feelings about trying for a natural birth. My first challenge was to find a doctor to assist me. I finally settled on one and made an appointment to talk to him. We decided that we could work together. I think both of us felt that we could trust the other to be open-minded and cooperative. I knew that whether he believed I could do it or not, he would do everything he could to help me succeed. Next, I knew that I would need to prepare well, so I looked for childbirth classes. I am so glad we chose the Bradley method. We were taught about optimum nutrition for our babies' development, exercises to prepare our bodies, how to relax through contractions, how to focus inward and work with our bodies to facilitate a faster, less painful birth, the stages of labor and the emotional signposts of each stage, and much more. We learned how to write a birth plan and to negotiate with the doctor and hospital about it. We wrote our plan and presented it to our doctor, discussing the things he was uncomfortable with, and came to a mutually agreeable plan. We took copies of our plan to the hospital with us so that the nurses would know what we wanted, also.*

— Kathryn S., Idaho

🍃 *Later in my pregnancy we took some very unusual birthing classes from a woman who worked with my midwife. The classes emphasized the emotions of the parents and helped us to look at our fears of the birthing process. I remember that my main fear was that my body would be permanently damaged by the birth. My husband's main fear was another c-section. She also had us explore different movements and vocal sounds that we could utilize in labor. She really opened my eyes to the fact that this was my labor, and that I had to find the unique way that my body gives birth. I still had my fear of failing, of having another c-section, but I felt ready for this birth.*

— Holly D., California

VBAC Support Groups

Although many childbirth instructors, midwives, and La Leche League leaders are helpful to women who want VBACs, the organizations and individuals in the United States who offer the most support are listed as follows. All of them can be found in the Resource Directory. They will provide you with information, support, and referrals to VBAC-friendly birth attendants, and they offer the most useful and up-to-date information about VBACs.

- International Cesarean Awareness Network (ICAN) probably has the most contact with women today. In addition to answering phone and mail inquiries, ICAN provides a newsletter and an Internet website with an e-mail address.

- Cesareans/Support, Education and Concern (C/Sec, Inc.), the oldest of the VBAC support groups, offers publications and referrals by mail and phone.

- Two individuals who have been VBAC counselors for decades are Nancy Wainer Cohen and Lynn Baptisti Richards. Both are authors and frequent VBAC lecturers.

❧ About the time I found out I was pregnant, I got a subscription to CompuServe at work and found the ICAN line on the Internet. It was the most important step in my VBAC process. Reading the stories of other women who had c-sections helped me realize that I still had a lot of unresolved feelings about my experience. I began to deal with my feelings of having missed out on the birth experience with my daughter and my fears of a repeat abruption. Through ICAN, I got information on doulas, and after my husband, Bob, and I interviewed several, we hired Kim. I believe she was instrumental in my successful VBAC. I can't thank ICAN enough for their support and encouragement. Even though I've never met these women, they helped make this happen for me. The outcome was great, but the process was the most empowering and important part of this journey.

—Alexandra G., Tennessee

❧ ❧ ❧

You have learned how to manage your fears, plan your VBAC, and find the right doctor or midwife, hospital or birth center. You appreciate what your helpers can do for you at the birth, and you know who they are going to be. Now it's time for the big day. The next chapter is all about a VBAC labor—how to prepare for it, and what to expect.

PART THREE

Giving Birth

❧ ❧ ❧

CHAPTER 8

Experience a VBAC Labor

A VBAC Labor
Nine Questionable Hospital Childbirth Procedures
Pain-Relieving Techniques for Labor

A VBAC LABOR is just like any other labor. An onlooker would not be able to tell the difference between you and a laboring woman who has not had a cesarean. If you haven't had a vaginal birth before, or you never got past 5 centimeters with previous labors, your VBAC labor will be like the labor of a woman having a vaginal birth for the first time, and like many other women having their first labor, your due date may pass before your labor begins. If you've gotten further along in the past, perhaps even to the pushing stage, your body will be more labor-experienced, like that of a woman who has previously given birth vaginally.

VBAC labors are, on average, a little longer than labors in general. If you had a cesarean for dystocia or prolonged labor, be prepared for a lengthy labor this time. But a past cesarean doesn't in itself lengthen the duration of labor. The factors that can cause labor to slow down (for example, if the baby is not in the most ideal position or if you have had an epidural) are the same for any first-time vaginal delivery, regardless of whether you've had a cesarean before.

There is always the chance of something unexpected happening, but certain things remain the same. The latent phase at the beginning of labor is always longer than transition, for example. And, unless your labor has been induced in some fashion, your baby will start labor for you.

A VBAC Labor

Some of the women who sent in their VBAC stories wrote that their cesareans, which had been for failure to progress or CPD, occurred because their labors did not progress at the rate of 1 centimeter an hour. Fifty years ago, when obstetrician Emmanuel Friedman wrote his analysis of the progress of labor, he could have had no idea his "Friedman curves" would be so misused. Decades later, he said, "There is no magic number of hours beyond which labor should not continue." A 1996 New Mexico study evaluating the length of labor found the average first labor to be 19.4 hours, and then 13.7 hours for a woman who had already had a vaginal birth. Yet 20 percent of the women studied had even longer labors. The standard that many obstetricians use, based, erroneously, on Friedman, is 12 hours for a first labor and 6 for a subsequent labor.

> ❧ *I really believe you can't fit a woman's labor into a textbook. I think it's probably normal for me to have a forty-hour labor, and not dilate for hours. For a doctor to say I must dilate 1 centimeter every hour is unbelievable. I think most doctors are too impatient today, knowing they have the means to interfere and end the process, and they are convinced it is less risky to do that, than to wait and let nature take its course.*
> — *Darla B., Washington*

The Latent Phase, or the Beginning of Labor. This is the least intense and the longest phase, ranging a few hours (rarely) in a woman with her first labor to twenty-four hours or more. (The early part of a VBAC labor, like any first labor, tends to be longer rather than shorter). Some women have early labor for days: while feeling mild contractions at irregular intervals, they pretty much go about their business, especially if they have other children who need their care. Called the latent phase, it's the beginning of the first stage of labor. At the end of the first stage, you will be fully dilated at 10 centimeters, but at the end of the latent phase, you'll be at 3 to 4 centimeters. Sometimes labor starts with the spontaneous breaking of the bag of waters. For some women, this speeds labor along, shortening the latent phase. For others, no contractions immediately follow. Some physicians recommend that women whose waters have broken at full term but who feel no contractions have their labors induced within 24 hours. This approach, however, can lead to another cesarean. Other physicians recommend waiting longer, since contractions usually start on their own within 48 hours after the breaking of the bag of waters. If your waters break before any contractions begin, be sure to call your doctor or midwife.

During the latent phase, you may feel mild contractions, menstrual-like cramps, indigestion, and/or diarrhea. If, however, your contractions are frequent and you're feeling lots of back pain, you should carefully read "Posterior Labor" on pages 142–43.

> ❧ *After arriving at the hospital, we tried every position for pushing for four hours. I really used two people, my husband and my doula, as one would hold me and the other would massage me. Finally, the doctor tried to turn the baby—who was posterior—manually, but that wasn't working. He offered forceps, and I agreed. So, we went to delivery, where my doctor turned the baby with the forceps, but then took them out so I could push him out with the next contraction. I pushed him out with such vocalization that the nurses gathered outside the door to see what was going on. He weighed 10 pounds. I was elated, but very sore. I wasn't sure the next day whether a vaginal birth was easier than a cesarean. I felt like I had been run over by a truck. But I was very proud of myself. My VBAC was in 1985.*
>
> — Denise C., Ohio

Sometimes women think the latent phase is just more Braxton-Hicks contractions—that is, frequent, mild, non-labor uterine tightening—or false labor. You may not know when you are in this phase, particularly if you had a previous posterior labor or if you're used to extremely painful menstrual cramps. You may think you're still in this early phase when in fact you're much farther along.

> ❧ *Labor began after 9:00 P.M. on January 25, 1989. I slept in between contractions, which were 10–20 minutes apart, until the morning. I knew I was in for a long haul. I went to the mall and walked. I showered, I ate lightly, I went into a friend's Jacuzzi. Sometime after 6:00 P.M. my labor*

🍃 Posterior Labor

You are experiencing "back labor" if you have short (30 seconds in duration), close (3 minutes apart or less), and painful contractions along with back pain that feels worse than the contractions. This happens when the baby is in a posterior position. It's not possible to determine if the baby is posterior by having his body felt through your abdomen. Listening to the heart tones is not a reliable way to tell, either. Your body has to tell you.

When labor is progressing slowly in the hospital, often the first actions taken are to break the amniotic sac and then administer some Pitocin. This is the worst thing for a posterior labor, because when the waters are broken, the contractions get stronger, and the baby's head starts to descend. For the baby to get from a posterior position into the ideal position for birth, his head must rotate up to 180 degrees (normally the head rotates 90 degrees or less). If the head descends too deeply before this rotation is accomplished, a vaginal birth is unlikely.

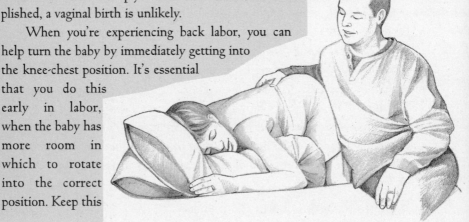

When you're experiencing back labor, you can help turn the baby by immediately getting into the knee-chest position. It's essential that you do this early in labor, when the baby has more room in which to rotate into the correct position. Keep this

support person came over and checked me. I was 3 centimeters dilated. I told her to go to her previously planned meeting and come back later, since it would probably be a while. My husband, Keith, and sister, Kim, were great. They walked with me, got me water, rubbed my back, and generally supported me. My contractions became closer, nearly 2 minutes apart. I still didn't want to leave for the hospital. My professional labor support person wasn't back yet, my water hadn't broken yet, and I thought I was probably only 3 centimeters dilated.

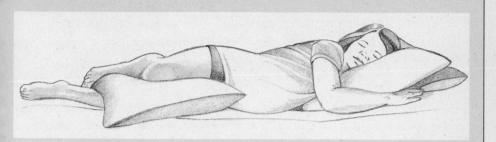

position until the contractions go to the front of your body and the back pain goes away. Have your helpers support you with lots of pillows and encouragement. You may find while you're in this position that the contractions become both more regular and more effective.

If the knee-chest position becomes too painful, try lying on your left side with one or two pillows under your jack-knifed right knee, and your left leg straight out and toward the back. This position can help the baby to rotate, too. Another advantage is that you can be attached to an EFM and an IV, if necessary. This is a good position for labor even if the baby isn't posterior.

You will know when the baby has turned, because you will feel so much relief. Sometimes turning the baby takes only a few minutes; sometimes it takes up to 45 minutes.

If the baby doesn't rotate early in labor, some doctors and midwives try to grasp the baby's head through the birth canal and rotate the head into the favorable anterior position. The only other recourse may be to offer the mother a paracervical block or an epidural. Without such interventions, it may be almost impossible for her to relax the deep muscles of her pelvic floor enough so that the baby can turn.

At 10:22 P.M. my contractions suddenly changed. I now felt pressure instead of pain—which is an indication that the baby will come soon. Needless to say, we left for the hospital. A few minutes later, my water broke in the car, and I could feel the baby's head descend. "Pull off the freeway now!" I said. "Now???" said Keith. As we pulled over to the off-ramp, a police officer showed up out of nowhere. "What seems to be the problem?" he asked. "Oh, nothing, my wife's just having a baby," said Keith, calmly. I think the officer almost had a heart attack. As Kim is videotaping, I am pushing. The paramedics (and firefighters and more police) show up within 2 minutes, just as the baby's head emerges. Another few pushes and the baby is born—it's a boy! They wrap him up and give him to me. I did it! I can't believe I actually did it!

— *April K., California*

Walk around, eat lightly, urinate often, and make yourself comfortable. At the end of this phase, your cervix will be opened to the width of 3 to 4 centimeters. If you can smile for the camera before you leave for the hospital, you're probably not at the end of this phase. In that case, just keep walking, either at your house or around the hospital parking lot, because that keeps your contractions strong and keeps your labor moving along. Remember: the hospital staff is prepared for women who are in *active* labor, at 5 centimeters or so. If you arrive at the OB floor at 1 or 2 centimeters, they'll either send you home, tell you to go walk somewhere, or put you in bed and give you Pitocin—which may have been the scenario with your cesarean labor.

❧ When my labor started, it was strong, progressive, and needed no induction or encouragement. I went about my day as planned, ate breakfast, walked, and I decided when it was time to go to the hospital. My doctor wanted me to call and come in as soon as labor started so I could be hooked up to the monitor and IV, but I didn't want to rush in and be strapped in bed. When I checked in, I was 6 centimeters. The doctor thought I was far enough along and going to "succeed," so he didn't hook me up! I did get a shot of a drug called Nubain, which helped me through a tough spot. I delivered vaginally an 8-pound, 14-ounce daughter after a total of seven hours of labor. I was so excited.

— *Jennifer S., California*

The Active Phase. Now labor is more intense, but it will not last as long as the first phase. Perhaps you'll have a "bloody show" now, a pink mucous discharge, although sometimes this appears before labor begins. (Don't confuse the bloody show with vaginal bleeding, which requires immediate medical attention.) You'll feel increasing backache and fatigue. More often than not, your membranes will rupture. Most of you will be at the hospital or birth center by now. If you're giving birth at home, your midwives will have arrived. Walk if possible, or at least change positions frequently, and rest between contractions. At the end of this phase, your cervix will be open to 6 or 7 centimeters.

> ❧ *Laurie checked me at 3:30 A.M. I was 6 to 7 centimeters dilated, and she was so encouraging by telling me the cervix was very soft and the baby's head was molding. If I could have thought clearly, I would have been elated to be further along than I ever had before. And the head was very low—obviously the baby [her fifth after four cesareans] had passed through my "funneled pelvis" and "flat sacrum." But I could not think clearly, and when Patrice reminded me how great it was that I was at 6 to 7 centimeters, all I could think of was how much I wanted to be complete. She reassured me that I sounded and acted just like every other laboring woman, and that, to me, made a big impact on my outlook. I guess I felt like I had this worse than any other woman alive, and to know that it is like this for others, too, helped me to accept it. From then on, I knew I was going to make it. I just prayed for it to be soon.*
>
> — Fae S., Michigan

> ❧ *As with my first labor, I spent much of my time in water—in this case, the bathtub. Instead of attempting to speed dilation by walking or nipple stimulation as I had the first time, I tried to conserve energy by resting between contractions. I anticipated another long labor. After fourteen hours of labor, I was at 4 centimeters, and certain I was going through transition. Judi told me I needed to pull myself together. She said, "It's going to hurt a lot worse before it gets better. You're not going to move forward with this unless you give in to it and accept it." And so I did. Six hours later I was at 7 centimeters, and we decided to try breaking my waters. That got me to 8. Someone told me later that the hardest part of labor in a VBAC is getting past the point where you "failed" previously. I found that to be the case. Getting past that magic 8 was rough.*
>
> — Heidi S., Virginia

Transition. This is the most intense phase of labor. Many women report their minds and bodies being in a different place during this time, especially if they are unmedicated. Contractions are very strong, seemingly continuous. At the end of this phase, you will finish the first stage of labor and be dilated at 10 centimeters. On average, it takes

15 minutes to an hour for the cervix to dilate the last three centimeters. You may feel rectal or lower back pressure. You may also feel warm and sweaty or chilled and shaky, and experience trembling, nausea, and perhaps vomiting. One of the markers of transition is sudden crabbiness. You may feel like pushing, but make sure you're fully dilated before you do—that is, at 10 centimeters.

> ✏ *After Leslie's water was broken this time, the contractions ceased for a while and then began again. However, they were not strong enough. I was reminded of her cesarean labor. Our doctor suggested using Pitocin to get Leslie over the edge. Leslie responded in a state of shock. "Really!" she said. She then turned to our doula and asked her what she thought. Debbie said, "No, let's try something else." We changed positions, and at the suggestion of the delivery-room nurse, we used nipple stimulation to intensify the contractions, and within 20 minutes we were at the pushing stage, and after 18 minutes of pushing, Leslie delivered a 9-pound baby boy. Leslie did not use any drugs or pain relief throughout the whole birthing process. Without our miracle-worker doula, Debbie, we could very easily have been headed down the road of Pitocin, epidural, and, ultimately, c-section.*
> — Jay E. and Leslie H., Illinois

Pushing. This can take as little as one push or as long as several hours. Unless you're anesthetized, you'll feel an overwhelming urge to push. If you had an epidural, you won't feel the wave of pushing urges because this anesthesia numbs you from the waist down. Instead you will be coached by your nurse or midwife to push. As the baby's head crowns, moments before birth, you may be told to pant or blow and to stop pushing. If you're not medicated, you may feel a stretching and stinging sensation in the vagina when the head crowns, and a tremendous sense of power and pleasure as the baby emerges from your body. Here's your baby!

> ✏ *To be honest, laboring without drugs, especially pushing, was hard and painful, but the euphoria after delivering was more than I expected.*
> — Karen V., Washington

Delivering the Placenta. After your baby is born, you will experience mild contractions for up to 30 minutes, and then the placenta, or afterbirth, will emerge. Most physicians shorten this time by pushing

> ### ✐ Practice Perineal Massage
>
> Perineal massage considerably reduces your risk for either a tear or an episiotomy. Prepare your perineum daily during the last month of your pregnancy. Get comfortable, and have your partner press freshly scrubbed fingers oiled with vegetable oil back and forth across the bottom part of your vagina, stretching enough to produce a slight tingling or burning sensation, for about 5 minutes each day. This massage makes your skin more elastic. You can do it yourself, too. Insert your thumbs as deeply as you can inside your vagina with your legs spread. Press the floor of the vagina down toward the rectum, and then press against the sides of the vaginal wall.
>
> During labor, midwives and some doctors will automatically support your perineum with warm, wet cloths when you're crowning, which also goes a long way toward reducing tears and the need for an episiotomy. Discuss the details of perineal massage with your doctor or midwife, and find out whether she will help support your perineum, too.

on the uterus to get the placenta to come out sooner. Midwives are more likely to let the placenta come out on its own. There's some evidence that waiting for the placenta to come out by itself reduces your risk for hemorrhage.

Checking the Scar. Since this is a VBAC, the dreaded, painful uterine exam to check the condition of the scar comes up about now. Studies have shown this exam to be unnecessary. (For more on this subject, see page 38.)

Nine Questionable Hospital Childbirth Procedures

If you've done your homework, you'll know that every hospital has certain procedures that are standard. Some of these procedures will be useful to you, and others will not. Most women undergo many of them, but none of them is 100 percent safe. Sometimes a procedure is performed because it's ideal for the mother; other times because it's routine at the hospital.

> ✎ *Nine Questionable Hospital Childbirth Procedures*
>
> 1. Shave
> 2. Enema
> 3. Making women lie flat on their backs during labor
> 4. Breaking the bag of waters
> 5. Intravenous attachment
> 6. Administration of Pitocin
> 7. Epidural anesthesia
> 8. Episiotomy
> 9. Vacuum extractor or forceps

You may not realize that you have the right at all times to refuse treatment of any kind from healthcare providers. Discuss all of these procedures with your birth attendant and hospital staff in advance. That way, when they're used on you, you'll know they were in your best interests, not just a matter of routine.

This list is organized in the order in which the procedures usually occur.

Shave. According to studies done in Baltimore sixty years ago and repeated in 1965 by researchers in Dallas, shaving the pubic hair for childbirth is an unnecessary discomfort. Some even suspect that shaving the genital area may increase a woman's chances of infection—usually from razor nicks that allow germs to enter. Although shaves are uncommon now, some hospitals do give them routinely. When you're calling hospitals to find those that are the most VBAC-friendly, ask if shaving is part of their routine.

Enema. Some people believe that administering an enema during labor serves to ease the baby through the birth canal by stimulating the uterus to contract, and that reduces the chances of fecal contamination. In 1982 a British research team found none of these claims to be true. Instead, it concluded that "such rectal assaults on women in labor should be discouraged." Bowels often empty on their own just prior to labor anyway. Most hospitals today don't give routine enemas, but some still do.

Making women lie flat on their backs during labor. This position can cause a drop in blood pressure, which affects the circulation of blood to the uterus. It depresses the baby's oxygen supply, decreases the intensity of contractions, and slows labor. Lying down makes it harder for the mother to push out both the baby and the placenta, since she is working against gravity.

The hospital staff may expect you to lie on your back if you are attached to an EFM—unless it's a telemetry EFM in a transmitter box that you can carry around in your pocket—and if you have an epidural or other medication. If you have an IV with Pitocin, you can walk around with support from your helpers.

If your cesarean was for failure to progress, you will especially want to avoid staying in bed for the duration of your labor. Walk, sit, lie on your side, get on your hands and knees, squat or stand with help from your supporters. Many women whose movement is unrestricted change positions frequently during labor.

❧ *With the baby's head fully applied to my cervix, everything changed. It was so intense all of a sudden! I got in the shower and thought all of those things that women think in labor: Why did I want to do this? Why does any woman do this? Why didn't I go and have that nice epidural? My contractions were not letting up: double-peaked and no time to rest in between. I began to feel like pushing after about an hour of those intense contractions. Lying down for a check was awful! I don't know how women can handle being in a bed during those contractions. I was moving, rocking, sitting on a birth stool, on the toilet, anything but lying down.*
— *Raven T., Indiana*

Breaking the bag of waters. Known as amniotomy, this procedure may shorten labor by 30 to 40 minutes or not at all. The disadvantage is that it removes the watery protection around your baby's head. Your bag of waters will always be broken if you have an internal EFM so that the probe can be inserted into your baby's scalp.

Intravenous attachment. The rationale for IV use is threefold: to give women the energy-producing calories of sugar water, to prevent dehydration, and to provide a ready hook-up when you need Pitocin or any other medication, or for an emergency, such as shock. But in an emergency, competent hospital staff can insert an IV quickly. IV needles can cause infections at the site of insertion. Furthermore, IV feeding as a substitute for food and fluids can lead to abnormal blood chemistry.

Some women find that a heparin lock is a good compromise. This is a needle inserted into the back of the hand. The needle has a plug on the end, which can be quickly inserted into an IV line if the need arises.

Some practitioners encourage light eating and drinking during labor—some broth, toast, and juice, for example. Check with your doctor or midwife to find out if your birth assistant can bring snacks along from home. Many doctors don't think eating and drinking, even lightly, is safe, because they think that food in the stomach will be vomited and breathed in, causing pneumonia, if you're given general anesthesia. But general anesthesia is rarely used today for childbirth. If general anesthesia does become necessary, the most important way to avoid a problem is to administer the anesthesia carefully, not to require fasting.

Administration of Pitocin. Oxytocin, a hormone that occurs naturally in the body, brings on labor. Pitocin, the synthetic version of that hormone, is used either to start labor or to speed it up. Contractions brought on by Pitocin are often much more intense than those that occur naturally. As a result, some women on Pitocin want an epidural for the pain. Among Pitocin's possible side effects are reduced blood flow to the baby during labor and an increased risk for jaundice in the newborn.

Other forms of induction commonly used in hospitals are membrane stripping (a rotating finger is inserted into the cervix, disconnecting some of the membranes from the lower part of the uterus) and amniotomy, mentioned earlier.

❧ *Then the waiting began. The last two weeks of my pregnancy seemed longer than the first eight and a half months. I knew I could ask for a cesarean at any time and have my baby in my arms. Only the memory of the repeat cesarean kept me from giving in to the temptation. As my deadline approached, I considered using castor oil to nudge me into labor, but*

❧ Home Remedies to Start or Speed Up Labor

If you are approaching your forty-second week of pregnancy and want to experiment with home remedies for delayed labor, you might try one or more of these methods. They have been used for ages to ripen the cervix (to soften and thin it), to induce labor, or both.

Sexual intercourse and orgasm. They cause the uterus to contract and oxytocin to be released in the bloodstream (Pitocin is the synthetic version of oxytocin). In addition, semen is a rich source of prostaglandins (the principal ingredient in the prostaglandin gel used in hospitals to induce labor).

Nipple stimulation. Whether in loveplay or in a hospital room, the gentle stimulation of one or both nipples also releases oxytocin, helping labor to either start or keep going. In one study, 84 percent of VBAC mothers who tried this technique managed to get their labors started with nipple stimulation.

Herbs. Although there is little published research on the use of herbs for labor, many midwives report that evening primrose oil, black or blue cohosh, gingerroot, birthroot, and red raspberry leaves brewed as tea are sometimes effective in either getting labor started or keeping it going.

Homeopathy. Among the most popular homeopathic remedies for late or slow labor are caulophyllum (or blue cohosh), cimicifuga, and pulsatilla. If you want to try these remedies, talk with a homeopathic physician or get a copy of *Homeopathic Medicine for Pregnancy and Childbirth*, by R. Moskowitz (North Atlantic Books, Berkeley, California, 1992).

Castor oil. Made from the bean of the castor plant, castor oil has a laxative effect, much like an enema. If the cervix is ripe already, castor oil can stimulate contractions. It apparently works best with women having their first labors. The usual dose is 2 ounces, and it ordinarily takes effect in two to six hours. Some midwives recommend an "induction mix" of 2 ounces each of castor oil, orange juice, and vodka. The best time to swallow castor oil is very early in the morning, so that you're not kept up at night with diarrhea.

Note: These techniques are described more fully by Lisa Summers in "Methods of Cervical Ripening and Labor Induction," *Journal of Nurse-Midwifery* 42(2), 1997.

decided to use my husband's help first. I told him that he helped get the baby in there; he could help get it out. "How am I supposed to do that?" he asked. "The same way you got it in there!" I responded. The prostaglandin in the semen seemed to do the trick. Saturday afternoon of Labor Day weekend my labor began, and continued for the next two days.

— Kathleen F., Ohio

Epidural anesthesia. Some women go into the hospital expecting not to use any drugs, but many others have planned all along to use all the painkillers offered. There are pain medications for early labor (1 to 5 centimeters dilation) and anesthesia for established labor (6 to 10 centimeters). The most popular labor medication in the United States, used by more than 90 percent of the women in some hospitals, is epidural anesthesia. With an epidural, an anesthetic is injected, usually by an anesthesiologist, into the lower spine, numbing the body from the waist down to the toes. When done correctly, the procedure usually provides excellent pain relief, and it can be a blessing for the exhausted laboring woman. Many hospitals are now offering "walking" epidurals that do not numb the legs, allowing the mother to get out of bed, go to the bathroom, and perhaps walk around a little.

❧ I had a new doctor and delivered at a different hospital. Throughout my pregnancy, my doctor kept telling me that our goal was to have a vaginal delivery. She said there was no reason why I shouldn't have one. When the day finally arrived, Dave and I went to the hospital prepared to have another cesarean, if necessary. It was another long labor. I opted for an epidural and felt great! I felt in control with the epidural. I felt clearheaded and able to make clear choices, whereas with my first pregnancy, I felt intimidated, even though I had taken all the childbirth classes. After eight hours in the hospital, it was time to push. I never got to the pushing stage with Lisa, so I really depended upon our nurse, Connie, to guide us through this process. After two hours, my doctor called in an OB for consultation because she thought I may need another cesarean. When the OB arrived, I had made some progress, but progress was slow. Twenty minutes later, he decided to use a vacuum extractor. Right away I noticed a difference and two pushes later, Hannah arrived! I wanted to tell everyone what it was like to push a child into the world!

— Nancy H., Washington

Since an epidural sounds so wonderful, why wouldn't every laboring woman want one? Because there are potential side effects for you and your baby. *No* drug administered during labor has been found to be totally safe for the baby, because all drugs cross the placenta into the baby's bloodstream. One of the most common effects on a baby during labor is a fluctuating heart rate. One of the most common effects on the mother is a drop in blood pressure. It's too soon to know if the walking epidural produces a different list of side effects.

About 14 percent of women develop fevers after having epidurals. This can affect their babies: A 1997 study found that one-third of the babies whose mothers developed fevers of 100.4 degrees or higher after birth are subjected to many tests and procedures. These newborns undergo painful tests for sepsis (an infection), because a fever can be an indicator of infection in the mother and, consequently, in her baby. The babies are taken to the neonatal intensive care unit to have blood drawn and, sometimes, to receive a lumbar puncture, a procedure in which fluid is removed from the spine. These babies are then kept in the hospital for up to three days, usually after their mothers have been discharged, and given antibiotics.

Another effect that an epidural can have on you is another cesarean, because epidurals, especially in a first-time labor—which is what you will be having if you have not had a previous vaginal birth—slow or stop labor. If you get an epidural when you're only 2 centimeters dilated, you have a 50 percent chance of having another cesarean. At 3 centimeters your chances are 33 percent, and 26 percent at 4 centimeters. If you wait until you're 5 centimeters dilated, an epidural will put you at no special risk for a cesarean.

🖉 *I was thinking of all those charts in the pregnancy books where each centimeter takes an hour, and from 1 to 4 centimeters if the contractions are this bad, from 4 to 7 the contractions are worse, and then there's transition where the contractions are unbearable. I didn't know how I would make it through worse contractions for six more hours. I wanted pain medication, and I wanted it now! They said I needed to wait until I was at 5 centimeters. As soon as I got back in the tub I could tell the contractions were getting more serious. I was begging for pain meds. The nurse said that the doctor and anesthesiologist would stop by my room on the way to do a c-section and I could have an epidural then. I was fully dilated at 10:30, and the baby was more than halfway down the birth canal. They told me it was time to push. My first thought was, "No way! I have to do this without help with the pain! This wasn't in my contract! I won't do it!" That thought was quickly brushed aside by Mother Nature. I was really glad once it was over that I hadn't had any pain meds.*

— Susan W., Washington

Although it's true that for some women an epidural can speed up labor, for most women an epidural lengthens labor, especially the pushing stage. If you get an epidural, you'll be attached to an EFM for the rest of your labor and will have your blood pressure monitored frequently (epidural use often brings a drop in blood pressure). Unless you have a walking epidural, you'll be confined to bed, meaning you'll probably need Pitocin to speed up your labor. (Sometimes it's the other way around: the increased pain due to the use of Pitocin can be the reason for the epidural.)

As the result of an epidural, you will probably also need either vacuum extraction or a forceps delivery, although you may be able to give birth without these aids if you're in a semi-sitting position instead of flat on your back. Chances are you'll also need a catheter to release urine in the immediate postpartum period. An unknown number of women have epidurals that don't completely take—a phenomenon called an anesthesia window—which can leave one side of the body with full sensation and the other side with no feeling. Numerous studies have discovered other possible side effects from epidurals to be depression, drowsiness, nausea, and vomiting; and, after birth, headaches, backaches, nausea, vomiting, shivering, and difficulty in urination.

Also, there is some evidence that you may be more susceptible to migraine headaches after having had an epidural during labor (although most women who have epidurals don't get migraines at all). A 1992 study from England shows a higher rate of migraines after childbirth among epidural users, especially those women who accidentally had dural punctures when the anesthesiologist missed the mark (the dura is the space in the spinal column next to the epidural space). If you have a family history of migraines, be sure to talk about this with your doctor or midwife while discussing epidurals.

Episiotomy. This is a cut made by a scissors in the tissue and skin that surrounds the vaginal opening and connects to the rectum (the perineum). It's usually made as the baby's head pushes against the perineum, thereby stretching it. Many doctors believe that this straight surgical cut to widen the birth canal will hasten labor and healing as well. It doesn't. Tears and damage happen more often and more severely with an episiotomy. An episiotomy doesn't shorten the pushing stage, either, although you might expect that it would.

About 65 percent of U.S. women have episiotomies, mostly with doctors. Midwives have far lower episiotomy rates because they recommend that women avoid giving birth flat on their backs; they encourage perineal massage before the baby is born; and they support the perineum with hot compresses when the baby is crowning. If you don't want an episiotomy, ask your doctor or midwife how often she makes this surgical cut, and what you can do in advance to avoid having an episiotomy.

Vacuum extractor or forceps. A vacuum extractor is a plastic cup that uses suction to "vacuum" the baby's head and help it move down the birth canal. It is less traumatic to the baby's head and to your bottom than forceps. Forceps are two large, metal, spoonlike blades (they look like salad tongs) that are inserted into the birth canal around either side of the baby's head to help it move down the birth canal. If you need either one of these procedures, you'll probably need an episiotomy as well. These tools are often used on women who have had epidurals.

Pain-Relieving Techniques for Labor

Labor pain occurs because uterine muscle contractions have to be very strong in order to move the baby down into the birth canal. Pain also comes from the pressure exerted by the baby's head as it widens the path to get through the canal. Much to many women's surprise, drugs, including epidurals, don't always relieve all of the pain of labor.

Whether you only want pain relief up until you can have an epidural at 5 centimeters, or you want to go all the way without drugs because your labor stalled when you had your epidural with your last birth or the drugs ruined your concentration the last time around, here are ten suggestions to shorten your labor, increase your birth pleasure, and reduce your pain.

🍃 *I got out some birth supplies and my "pain bag" with all my gadgets in it. I turned on all the lights and the radio because it had been too dark and quiet for me the last time I was in labor. I took a hot shower and then labored on the bed, listening to the radio for distraction. I kept a hot pad on my back and squeezed a comb in my hand, which felt good. I also would roll the tennis ball against my lower back when I had back pain. I also found myself saying the alphabet in my mind for distraction, which seemed to help, so I kept doing it. Counting objects was one of the things listed in Adrienne Lieberman's book [Easing Labor Pain, Harvard Common Press, 1992], which sounded silly at the time but worked for me. Scott came in every once in a while to give me ice water, but it was harder to concentrate when he came in, plus he had to deal with the kids, so he didn't stay long.*

— Linda G., New York

🍃 *I knew it was all up to me. I mentally prepared myself for another long labor. Some of the things I gathered were tennis balls, a heating pad, and a rolling pin, which can all be used for back labor. I also got some combs for squeezing, lollipops for a dry mouth, and I compiled a list of suggestions and inspiring statements that I planned to tape on the wall and stare at when things got tough. I exercised a lot during this pregnancy. I did low-impact and step aerobics until my fifth month and then walked. I kept telling myself that labor is a physical event and that I need to be in shape. [She had a VBAC this time after two cesareans.]*

— Kelly L., Virginia

Take warm baths or showers. This is the favorite form of pain relief for many laboring women. Have someone help you sit or stand. Get into a Jacuzzi, if you're lucky enough to have access to one. Warm water can not only speed up a labor, but it can take the edge off the pain. Water makes it easier for you to reduce your inhibitions and "allow" labor to happen.

🍃 *Ten days past my due date I woke with mild contractions. I was 2 centimeters when I arrived and we realized we were in for a long haul. By* noon the contractions were stronger and I was really working through them. At 2 P.M. I got into the whirlpool bath where it was wonderful: the heat was great, and the calm atmosphere really helped. At 3 P.M. they took me out of the bath to give me drugs, but on examining me my doctor said I was at 10 centimeters—so no drugs. As the head crowned the doctor saw that the baby's fist was right next to her cheek. She pushed her own hand in and pulled out the baby's arm. The baby was delivered like the Statue of Liberty, with one arm over her head. Tara weighed 9 pounds, 11 ounces.

— Wendy A., Quebec, Canada

🍃 I ate normally the whole time during my labor. Forty hours later, on Saturday night, contractions were sporadic—3 minutes, 7 minutes, 2 minutes, et cetera. When I was checked, I was dilated 7 centimeters. I had no real pain up to this point. I was feeling contractions a little more, so my midwife put me in the tub. Wonderful! I loved the water; there was no pain at all. Judy came one and a half hours later and checked me. I was 10 centimeters and did not know it.

— Jennifer M., Pennsylvania

Try cold packs or hot packs for back pain. Cold cloths on the back or forehead, especially during transition, can be helpful, as well as ice packs if you have back labor. The numbing effect of cold packs slows

---

🍃 *Pain-Relieving Techniques for Labor*

- Take warm baths or showers.
- Try cold packs or hot packs for back pain.
- Encourage your supporters to be your natural tranquilizers.
- Get in a position that feels good.
- Try a massage or a backrub.
- Listen to relaxing, soothing music.
- Use visualization to reduce the pain.
- Make your hospital room more homelike.
- Try TENS (transcutaneous electrical nerve stimulation) or a birthing ball.

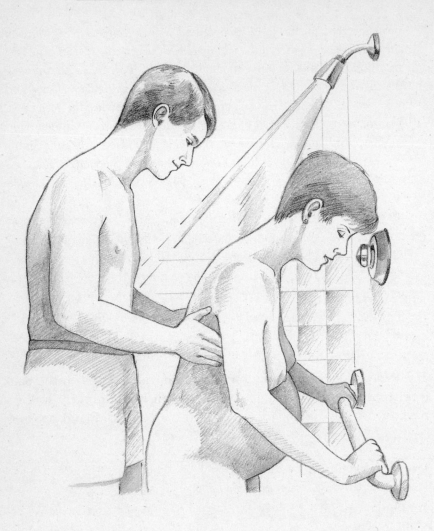

the transmision of pain impulses. Warm washcloths and electric heating pads are helpful for some women, too.

Encourage your supporters to be your natural tranquilizers. Ask your partner and your birth assistant to give you only positive reinforcement. Labors and laboring women thrive on encouraging words. Make sure they both have a list of things to do to help reduce your pain. The very presence of your supporters will reduce your pain and shorten your labor.

Get in a position that feels good. It could be sitting, lying on one side, kneeling, standing, moving into a supported squat (with someone supporting you under your arms so that you don't have to hold yourself up), getting on the bed on all fours—or all of these. Women who have freedom in labor to change positions do so an average of seven times. Staying upright—whether walking, standing, or kneeling—often helps speed along a labor, too. Experienced birth attendants know that you'll find your best pain-reducing position on your own. If you're feeling heavy back labor that feels worse than the contractions, immediately get into a knee-chest position until the pain moves around to the front of your body. (See "Posterior Labor" on pages 142–43.) When you are approaching the pushing stage, squatting may feel good and may also hasten the birth.

Try a massage or a backrub. Tell your helpers where it feels best to apply pressure. Strong force applied to a spot on the lower back during contractions using the "heel" of the hand is often helpful. You could also have someone give you a foot and ankle massage. Pressing on the acupressure point just behind the ankle bone can provide a lot of relief.

Listen to relaxing, soothing music. Bring along a radio or a tape or CD player with earphones. This isn't for every woman, but those who like it believe it shortens labor.

Use visualization to reduce the pain. As mentioned in Chapter 2 (see the meditation instructions on page 43), visualization is seeing in your mind's eye a desired goal as if it's already happened. During labor, visualize your baby coming out the birth canal. Imagine each contraction pulling the baby down and out through your body. If you practiced meditation during your pregnancy, especially the mental exercise of going to a favorite place, it will serve as a useful skill during labor.

🌿 *When she was weighed, our estimated 8¹/₂ pound baby was actually 9 pounds, 15¹/₂ ounces and 22 inches long. We were all amazed, and glad it was over. Reflecting back, several things stick out in my mind that helped me reach my goal of having a VBAC. The first was my intense desire and*

Positions that feel good

1. Sitting with the support of a helper.

2. Sidelying with the support of your partner or your labor assistant. Many women switch sides periodically while using this position, especially if they are trying to turn a baby who is posterior.

3. Kneeling. This woman's partner is pressing his hand firmly in the triangle area right above her buttocks to relieve her lower back pain. She is squeezing the hand of her birth assistant, another pain-relieving technique. Her birth attendant is also probably "breathing" with her, helping her with visualization, or giving her words of encouragement, such as "You can do it" or "You sound great." Women often say that verbal encouragement is the most important form of support they received during labor.

4. Standing and leaning with help. Your supporters can help you walk during labor, too. If you have an IV, one of your helpers can pull along the IV stand as you walk.

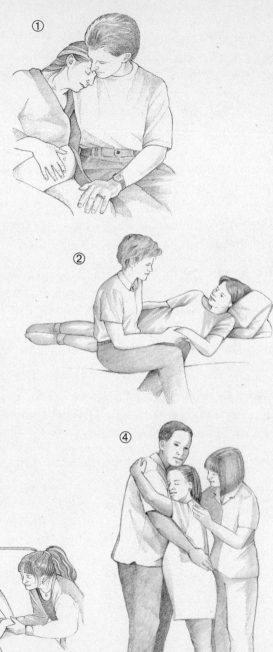

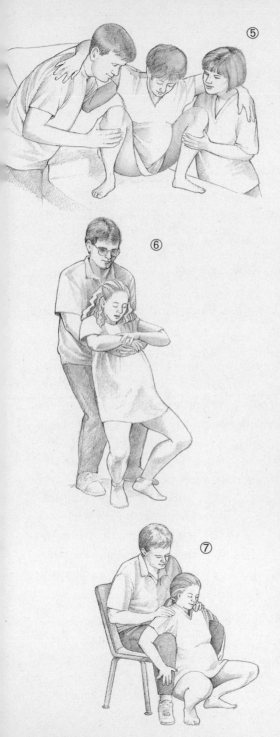

Since squatting both speeds labor and relieves pain, it's a good idea to know several ways to squat as you near the pushing stage. Experiment with your supporters to find the right squatting position for you. Here are three examples. Other versions of squatting require the use of a squatting bar or holding on to a chair, railing, or bedside.

5. Squatting on the bed with a supporter on either side. *This squat is often used during the pushing stage, and even by moms who have had light epidurals. The birth bed is placed in the recliner position, with the head of the bed tilted upright at an angle, and the foot of the bed extending out horizontally. The mother leans back into the "recliner" to rest between contractions. Her partner stands on one side of the bed and a support person on the other. When a contraction begins she wraps one arm around her partner and the other around her support person, and they lift her forward into a squat. When the contraction is over, they ease her back into the recliner to rest.*

6. Standing supported squat. *Known as "Odent style," this squatting position was popularized by pioneering French childbirth physician Michel Odent and his midwives in Pithiviers, France. Its advantage for the laboring woman is that she doesn't have to use any effort to support herself. It can, however, be a difficult position for a helper to maintain for a long time.*

7. Squatting, supporting herself with her arms on the thighs of her seated partner. *In this squat, the partner is seated on a chair. The mother stands in front of him, between his legs. When a contraction begins, she squats and supports herself by placing her forearms on his thighs.*

*sheer determination to deliver vaginally. I actually visualized myself hav-
ing a successful VBAC.*

— *Heidi O., Washington*

Make your hospital room more homelike. Wear your own clothes during labor, if you want to. There's no rule stating that you have to wear
a hospital gown, though a nurse may say there is. Bring a favorite
thing or two from home to make your room truly more homelike—
pictures of your other children, mementos, and so on.

**Try TENS (transcutaneous electrical nerve stimulation) or a birthing
ball.** TENS applies controlled, mild electrical stimulation to the skin
by means of electrodes attached to the skin with conducting gel. A
laboring woman controls where she puts the TENS unit. The pain
relief comes from the buzzing sensation, which provides a competing
sensation to the labor pain. There is no evidence that TENS causes
any harm to mother or baby, and many women find it very effective
during labor.

A birthing ball is a large ball originally developed for use in physical therapy. It allows women to change positions easily, and doesn't
lose its shape like a bean bag does. With knees slightly apart, women
sit and automatically rock on the balls, providing gentle pelvic movement that helps their babies get into the ideal position for birth. The
use of the birthing ball reduces labor pain, including back pain.
Women find that sitting on a birthing ball is far more comfortable
than sitting on chairs, beds, or toilet seats. It can be used on the floor,
the bed, or in the shower—a boon for women who want the pain relief
of water during labor, but who don't want to stand in the shower.

Although the birthing ball and TENS are commonly used in
Europe to alleviate childbirth pain, they are rarely offered to laboring
women in the United States. If you want to try either option, ask your
childbirth educator for more information.

*✎ I tried the TENS machine, which was far more helpful than I expect-
ed. TENS is commonly used here in England in the early stages of labor. If
I remember correctly, I put the pads on my back and it produced a tingling
sensation which distracted me from the labor pains. I actually kept the
things on right through to the end, and my husband and Caroline, the mid-*

wife, took turns pressing the buttons when the contractions came on. I had been doing it myself in the beginning but as things intensified, I got very involved with breathing and moaning and Caroline suggested that they could do it to help out. Gave us all something to do! The people who hire them out advertise in all the maternity hospitals and childbirth-oriented magazines.

— Helen K., England

❧ *When the contractions started to get stronger, the best position for me to be in was on my knees resting my upper body on a physical therapy ball. I had front and back labor. An ice pack on my back felt great! I went to the bathroom as soon as we got to my hospital room and I had bloody show. I really felt good because I knew things were progressing—something that didn't happen with my cesarean labor with Garrett. I continued to lean on the ball either in bed or standing. Sally, my midwife, asked if I wanted to go into the tub. I said yes. So we headed two doors down the hall. The tub was small, and though it didn't feel great to sit in it, it had a little ledge that pressed against my back. That and being in the water felt good. Sandy, my doula, stayed with me the whole time giving me ideas for dealing with pain—the best one was to really focus on relaxing my bottom and saying "relax" or "open" during contractions.*

— Jill L., Washington

❧ ❧ ❧

No matter how short or long your labor, and no matter how your baby was born, whether vaginally or by cesarean, your VBAC labor is over. And your baby is born. Congratulations! The next, and final, chapter in this book gives tribute to all of you who have given birth, along with suggestions for those of you who are having another cesarean.

CHAPTER 9

⬿ ⬿ ⬿

Appreciate Your Birth Experience

Appreciating Your VBAC Experience
If You Have a Planned Repeat Cesarean
If You Have an Unplanned Repeat Cesarean

NOW THAT I'm down to my last words on the subject of VBACs, I want to share a few more women's stories with you, stories that show birth's unpredictability and disappointments along with the parts of it we always treasure. Some of these women did everything right and still didn't get their VBACs. Others, including two from the same town in Ohio, received unexpected benefits and personal power from having both: one a cesarean and one a VBAC. Two are stories of sadness because babies died. And a mom who had her first VBAC in the 1970s gives us a story of hope for the future.

The last part of this chapter is a list of suggestions for an "ideal" repeat cesarean for those of you who won't be having a VBAC this time. I close with comments for those of you who discovered in labor that your VBAC plans would not work out.

Appreciating Your VBAC Experience

⬿ *As with all VBACs, it starts with the birth of my first daughter and the cesarean. I cannot blame the cesarean on outside variables, on a hurried doctor wanting to make a golf game, or a wrong diagnosis, or no support. I believe things have to happen for a reason, and I would not be in the* place I am in my life now without the experience of the cesarean. I was shocked, confused, and felt completely defeated about the birth. Every birth takes you to a place you have never been before, and I know that I didn't want to visit that place the cesarean took me ever again. I grieved for all the losses this birth gave me. Although my daughter was the most precious gift, it would take the healing of my next experience to make me appreciate what a gift birth is.

— Kristin M., Indiana

❧ Looking back, I am grateful for all my birth experiences—especially my cesarean. If not for that birth, I would not be the person I am today. It changed me in more ways than I can mention. A birth such as my first VBAC would not be acceptable to me now, but at the time it was the most empowering experience of my life. I have grown and expected more of myself and my births since then, but it was that experience that allowed this metamorphosis.

— Sunday T., Ohio

❧ I felt like I had conquered the world. After two other tries, I felt like I had achieved the birth that I wanted. I felt strong, brave, and powerful. Aside from my wonderful emotional high, I couldn't believe how good I felt physically. My VBAC was one of the most empowering events of my life. It was so wonderful that since then I have become a doula. I feel that one of my roles in life is to help women to make good choices for themselves surrounding the birth process. Birth can be a life-altering event. I want to help other women to make that event a positive one.

— Jamie S., Ohio

❧ Now that my VBAC has been almost a whole year ago, I am enjoying new feelings of being a part of that group of people known as "women who have delivered a baby." Yes, the feelings are new, even after having four children by cesarean previously. I didn't feel cheated or odd in any way before the VBAC, but afterwards I felt as if I had finally arrived at womanhood.

— Fae S., Michigan

❧ I pushed myself farther than I thought possible. I feel the VBAC homebirth gave me back the control I had lost at my first birth. And it gave me *real confidence as a person and in my abilities as an intuitive parent. The VBAC for me was an incredibly empowering experience.*

— Megan W., Washington

❧ *I had the most beautiful childbirth experience, and for the first time one of my daughters was present. I shared with my beloved husband and my sixteen-year-old girl the birth of a beautiful little girl. When she was born, she had a very hard time trying to breathe by herself. And despite the doctor's efforts and intensive care technology, she couldn't make it and only lived for an hour. This was the hardest pain I had ever had, and I was unable to understand why she left so soon. After several days of crying and trying to accept that my baby had passed away, I began to realize she had accomplished her mission in this world because my family became more loving and united than ever. My teenagers could see how life is a great gift that deserves respect and awe. I also learned that God Almighty is the only one that gives life and decides when it is over.*

When I think of her, my memories are those of a birth in which I worked and did my best. I thank God I was free of drugs and had a normal vaginal birth, because I was able to feel the magical moment of her birth and also to hold her and kiss her and welcome her to the world. I also had the strength to hold her and kiss her goodbye, giving me the opportunity to see and believe she had really died. This helped me and all my family very much to accept death joyfully as part of life. I am also very glad I had a VBAC because the pain in my soul was so deep, and the pain in my breasts was so hard to bear, it was a very good thing I didn't have to recover from surgery, too.

— Gabriela O., Mexico

❧ *It had been twelve years since I had a cesarean and years since I had given birth in a hospital. Even though we knew we needed to be in the hospital, it was a very difficult way to labor. I labored for twelve hours before they finally did the cesarean. I still firmly believe that women can and should give birth naturally and that homebirth is a safe and wonderful way to give birth, but I now have a new level of looking at the whole picture. I have always felt that I would be willing to sacrifice my "experience" for the health of my baby, as I believe most women would. This cesarean had a completely different feeling for me than my previous two. I willingly sub-*

mitted myself to the surgery for the life of my baby. My focus was solely on what was best for him.

I feel that the most important thing for women having VBACs is that they feel they have made the best choices and decisions. It was important to me that I didn't feel like I gave in to having a cesarean. I have been attending births as a birth assistant for the past four years and it has been my experience that even if women don't end up with the birth of their dreams or even a VBAC, they can leave their births happy and satisfied if they feel that they made informed choices and had the opportunity to try everything possible to avoid a cesarean and other interventions. Now that I have experienced the death of one of my children, there is new meaning to the bottom line being a healthy baby.

— Michele F., Virginia

🖋 I had a cesarean in 1974 for an abrupted placenta. That was a pretty hairy experience as my baby was born about two months prematurely. All worked out well, though, and college graduation is behind that tiny kid (2 pounds, 10 ounces) now. I had my first vaginal birth in 1978, which made me a pioneer in my community. After much searching and discouragement, my first vaginal birth happened in a hospital without any interventions whatsoever. I did it!

Following that birth I went on to plan four more births at home. Each, of course, was memorable and full of anecdotes. One of the most interesting aspects of births number 3 and number 4 is that we had a dear friend who was an OB who had never done a homebirth, but was game to come along and work with a CNM and, in birth number 4, a lay midwife, too. What was wonderful was that they were all there for me. Each person shared knowledge willingly and felt comfortable with the others. That gave me hope for the future—of a cooperative birth system.

— Jane S., New Jersey

If You Have a Planned Repeat Cesarean

This book is dedicated to having a successful VBAC, but few birth professionals report that 100 percent of the women in their care who want VBACs have them. Some of those women share their feelings about that in this section.

Even though you may want a VBAC, you may discover in advance that it won't be possible because, for instance, your baby is in a persistent breech position. Or perhaps, after reading this book, you realize a VBAC is not for you—for any number of reasons. Don't give up on some of the things you want, though, just because you're not going to have a VBAC. Here are ways to help you get what you want and to plan the "ideal" repeat cesarean. Planning can make all the difference.

❧ *After having my firstborn, I could have been handed a cabbage [instead of] my baby. I didn't care. I was either in pain or drugged. My doctor may have been a skillful surgeon, but he was terrible with the emotions of a new mother. During my pregnancy, I mentioned that my husband wanted to be at the birth. I mentioned bonding, too. "Bonding!" he scoffed. "Bonding is for ducks. You're not having a duck, are you?" My second child's birth three years later was 100 percent different. I had a doctor who believed in bonding (but not VBACs). I saw my daughter as she emerged from me— they held the green sheet aside. She was bloody and beautiful. My husband was there taking pictures; so were the nurses. It was a completely loving and wonderful experience.*

— Marlene C., California

Choose a doctor with lots of cesarean experience. And make sure it's someone whose operating room philosophy is the same as yours (you want to see the birth and have your helpers with you, for example). It's always true that surgical outcomes are better with physicians who have lots of experience in the surgery you will have. Some of you will be having your cesareans in hospitals where obstetric residents (doctors who are still in training) sometimes perform cesareans. When you can, avoid them for your surgery. They have less experience with cesareans than doctors who are out in practice. Ask the doctors whom you are considering about their average postpartum cesarean infection rate; they will have some idea. Check with hospital nurses and childbirth educators for these answers, too. There are many reasons for postpartum cesarean infections (see Chapter 1), including the complications that may have brought about the cesarean, and the health of the woman, but some infections can be linked to individual surgeons' techniques and their practices in the operating room.

⬚*If You Have a Planned Repeat Cesarean...*

- Choose a doctor with lots of cesarean experience.
- Find a physician and a hospital that are prepared to perform surgery only when you have gone into labor.
- Have every step of the cesarean and the preparation for it explained to you.
- Arrange for regional anesthesia.
- Review the possibility of a blood transfusion with your doctor.
- Make sure you can have your partner or your labor assistant in the operating room.
- Ask about your personal operating room preferences.
- Request to hold your baby as soon as possible and have the baby examined near you.
- Arrange to feed your baby as soon as possible.
- Plan to have daily help both in the hospital and at home.
- Consider new ways of coping with post-surgical pain and discomfort.

Find a physician and a hospital that are prepared to perform surgery only when you have gone into labor. Some doctors or hospitals prefer to give drugs to stop labor or to schedule your cesarean weeks before your due date. Since the 1980s there's been a consistent decrease in weekend births, and for repeat cesareans the number of Sunday births has plummeted. Most cesareans, whether first or repeat, occur Monday through Friday. If you want to schedule your cesarean, there are advantages to planning it for your due date, or after, so that you reduce the risk for prematurity. Babies born by cesarean are, on average, smaller and born after fewer weeks of gestation, although this statistic is no doubt affected by the need for emergency cesareans. If you go into labor on your own, however briefly, you'll still give your baby some of the advantages he would get from a vaginal birth. In particular, you'll reduce his risk for a stay in the high-risk nursery by increasing his level of catecholamines (labor hormones), which help prepare your baby to live outside the womb.

❧ My daughter was breech. Though the doctors wanted to section me two weeks before my due date, I refused, believing there was always a chance she would turn in labor. But she didn't. After nine hours of labor, I was 6 centimeters dilated. She was in a single breech position doing a split with one foot over her shoulder and the other down into the vagina, which is what was giving me the powerful urge to push. I knew I had done all I could and agreed to the cesarean. I also requested that there be no screen in front of me, so I could see her coming out. Her birth was a beautiful birth for me because all decisions were my own.

— Cathy D., New Jersey

Have every step of the cesarean and the preparation for it explained to you. This will help to increase your understanding and reduce your anxiety, no matter what your cesarean experience was the last time. Even though you've had a previous cesarean, techniques change and options vary from doctor to doctor and from hospital to hospital. Knowing what to expect always reduces pre-surgery anxiety. The more you know about what will happen, the more influence you will have on the events. If possible, interview your anesthesiologist in advance, too. If you're having an emergency cesarean, you'll get whichever anesthesiologist is on call, but if you're having a planned cesarean, even one that starts with some labor, you might have a choice on which anesthesiologist will be there.

Arrange for regional anesthesia. Sometimes there are valid reasons for general anesthesia, including an "epidural window"—that is, when some part of the epidural doesn't take and a woman can feel the pain of surgery. But most of the time, regional anesthesia—often epidurals and spinal blocks—is ideal. The mother has fewer side effects with regional anesthesia and is awake when her baby is born. Regional anesthesia has become the standard in the United States for cesareans, but some anesthesiologists may prefer other approaches. Just as you need to find a surgeon with lots of experience to perform your cesarean, ideally you will be able to find a board-certified anesthesiologist who has lots of experience with the regional anesthesia you want, and prefers it, too. If your regional anesthesia the last time left you with ongoing back pain or headaches, ask about other options.

Review the possibility of a blood transfusion with your doctor. Up to 10 percent of women who have cesareans need blood transfusions. Ask your doctor how she makes her decision for a transfusion—there is no standard rule, and different doctors and hospitals have different regulations. If you know well in advance that you will have a cesarean, discuss with your doctor the option of donating your own blood. This is especially important for women who have suspected placental problems, which often cause hemorrhaging. Although there is no 100 percent reliable way to test for diseases in blood products, the reasons for considering donating your own blood go beyond avoiding the risk for HIV, hepatitis, and other blood-borne diseases. Each person has a blood print as unique as a fingerprint. The safest blood to use for a transfusion is your own because you can avoid weakening your immune system, as can potentially happen when any foreign substance is introduced into the body, from allergens and cold germs to someone else's blood. The way this process is done in obstetrics apparently poses no threat to your unborn baby, but discuss it with your doctor. Your physician will give you guidelines on how much this might cost (be sure and check with your insurance company—see Chapter 4 for more information), and you can plan ahead so that you can accumulate a sufficient amount of blood in the time you have between donating it—usually in the ninth month—and your operation.

Make sure you can have your partner or your labor assistant in the operating room. He or she can serve as your advocate, and will be able to tell you later on about everything that happened in detail. Times have changed from the days when most fathers weren't permitted in the operating room for a cesarean; now their presence is far more common. But it's important to check anyway, because it's a decision made by individual doctors and hospitals.

Some women want both their partner and their labor assistant with them, even when the surgery is scheduled and no labor takes place. If you want both, ask. They can give you details on the cesarean. Even if you are awake and the screen is down, you still can't see everything or absorb all that is happening. Remember, all women have a need to discuss their births. It's part of the transition to new motherhood, even when you have other children. Since ideally someone will accompany the baby to the nursery, having a second person there means that the other person can stay with you.

Ask about your personal operating room preferences, including taking photos or videos or playing music. It's important to many women to personalize their births no matter where they occur. This may be true with you, too. Do you want one of your helpers to take photos or a video? If so, you need to find out in advance if it's okay, and when, where, and how it should be done. Do you want to listen to particular music on headphones during the operation? If you do, you'll need someone to help you with the headphones while you're on the operating table. Some women even arrange for their music of choice to be played in the operating room during the cesarean, if the doctor and staff agree. A Pennsylvania mother who sent in her VBAC story wrote that she brought along a tape of Handel's *Messiah,* which was played in the cesarean operating room as her daughter was born.

Request to hold your baby as soon as possible and have the baby examined near you. If your baby is healthy, and you've had regional anesthesia, there's often no good argument for *not* doing this. You will need help, however, in holding the baby because you will be flat on your back—another reason to have your helpers nearby. Ask if your baby could be examined on a nearby table that is within your view, or, if the baby's examining table is portable, ask that it be moved to a place where you can see your baby's exam.

Arrange to feed your baby as soon as possible. Whether you are breastfeeding or bottlefeeding, you and your baby will benefit from the earliest possible contact. If you are breastfeeding, you will help bring in your regular milk sooner and avoid potential breastfeeding problems. If you're going to feed your baby as soon as possible, you will need help (yet another reason for your own helpers). Hospital nurses often don't have the time to do something that you want when you want it, and they welcome patients who bring their own assistants.

Plan to have daily help both in the hospital and at home. It's not reasonable to rely on the hospital staff every time you want to move, get up, or hold and feed your baby. Sometimes people recovering from surgery think that because they or their insurance company are paying an average of $941 a day for their stay, those kind of prices mean that someone on the hospital staff will be at their beck and call. This is not the case. Furthermore, help in the hospital is not enough. After a stay of several days, you will go home, still many weeks and months away from full recovery. Now is the time to ask friends and family for help. Don't be bashful. You're not only recovering from surgery, but you have a newborn with twenty-four-hour needs. Enlist a friend to arrange for others to cook simple meals and handle easy chores. Call your church or synagogue and ask if they have a program to help new mothers. If you can, hire a professional postpartum doula who will come in and do housework, childcare, and cooking, and help you with the baby. Some services are covered by insurance. (The "Mother-Helpers" section in the Resource Directory lists organizations that can give you local referrals. You can check ads in your local parenting publications, too.)

Consider new ways of coping with post-surgical pain and discomfort. Typically, women who have cesarean surgery receive numerous drugs before and during the operation, as well as many later on for pain relief and to reduce the risk of infection. Part of the reason some women experience depression after a cesarean is that it is a side effect from the combination of drugs they are taking. Nausea and vomiting are common, too.

In a 1996 study, continuous pressure on the Neiguan point (on the inside of the wrist, about three finger-widths up from the wrist fold in the midline between two tendons) substantially reduced the nausea and vomiting that are associated with epidural morphine, which is administered for post-cesarean pain. The easiest way to put pressure on this point is with anti-nausea wristbands—sold under the brand names Morning Garde, Sea Band, and Acuband—or similar products. These stretchy bracelets, which apply light pressure to the Neiguan point, were originally developed to prevent motion sickness and seasickness. You can use one or two bands, and wear them all the time or just when you feel nauseated. Press the button on each band every half hour or so, using a circular motion for greater effect.

Another non-drug pain reliever is transcutaneous electrical nerve stimulation, or TENS (see page 162), which helps you get your mobility back sooner. Research suggests that it's difficult for nurses to know what your level of postpartum pain is, so it's not only up to you to say what you feel but to have non-drug options as well.

> ✎ *The next three babies (after three earlier cesareans) were born while my husband was in the military. I had relatively positive experiences with babies number five and six because we were blessed to be placed in Family Practice, where I had the same doctor throughout pregnancy and delivery. With these two babies, I learned how to go completely without pain medication after the surgery. I used a TENS unit, a device that is used in physical therapy. No one had used it for surgical pain before, to our knowledge, but it worked great for me. I would much rather be in a little bit of pain than be groggy from the drugs. I believe this helps with a better recovery, also.*
>
> — *Kathryn S., Idaho*

If You Have an Unplanned Repeat Cesarean

Your plans for a VBAC probably didn't change until you were in labor. Then the unexpected happened, and you didn't have time to plan for an "ideal" repeat cesarean. You always knew that a cesarean was a possibility, but you didn't think it would happen to you. You're disappointed, but you're probably not devastated because you gained personal strength from all the effort you put in for a VBAC birth. You knew you did everything you could to have a VBAC. This birth may not have happened the way you expected, but all your careful planning and decision making are not for naught. Your baby has benefited from your efforts and your thoughts. Nothing can take away from that.

Appreciate your feelings, and talk about them with others—if not with family and friends, then through support groups such as ICAN and C/Sec (see the Resource Directory).

> ✎ *I know now what it actually feels like both physically and mentally to give birth in different ways. Although the last birth was the easiest, they all were precious; each had its good points and bad points. I can understand*

a woman's disappointment if the birth experience doesn't go as planned, but this does not make the baby any less precious at the end of it. I try to encourage women and men to debrief their labors afterwards, the good points and the bad points, with their partners to help bring it all into perspective. I also try to tell them that their labors may not go as planned and to have a contingency plan, and if this does happen that it is all right to be disappointed, and not to feel guilty about this. My experiences have taught me this and I feel I can give a better view of birth now than before I had children.

— Jocelyn C., midwife, England

❧ I attempted a VBAC in 1988. We had tried to set things up for success by taking special VBAC childbirth classes and by hiring a midwife to labor with me until it was time to go to the hospital. When labor did not progress much, the midwife started playing head games with me—"You should be thinking about why you don't want this baby to come out"— and suggested breaking my waters and setting up an IV drip on the living room sofa to combat my dehydration. This was a signal to me to get over to the hospital. I was shocked to hear that the OB's evaluation of how far along I was bore no resemblance to the midwife's, and that in fact I was getting nowhere. I had an epidural, followed two hours later by a repeat cesarean. We were devastated to have put all that energy and suffering into a hopeless cause, but we sure were happy to see Sky—all 10 pounds and 2 ounces of him! You can truly make your best effort at VBAC and still fail. We seem to have this idea that we can control birth and get the experience we want. If you fail, it isn't because you didn't try enough.

— Nellie S., New York

❧ I had five cesarean births: my first in 1975, my last in 1989. I had general anesthesia with the first three and epidural with the last two. I had both external and internal classical incisions. Through the years I studied and read everything I could find about birth, cesareans, VBAC, et cetera. I started support groups, advocated for changes in hospital policy, and much more. But I couldn't find anyone to "allow" me to have a VBAC. I finally reconciled; unfortunately, I couldn't have a VBAC. In the past six years I've apprenticed with midwives and have attended over 150 births. I am a doula and doula trainer, Birthworks childbirth educator, Joyful

*Child parenting teacher, and am starting the Arizona ICAN chapter soon.
I've helped a lot of women with their birth experiences, but never applied
any of it to myself.*

— *Rhonda H., Arizona*

❧ ❧ ❧

Kiss your partner and that new baby. They need reassurance, too.
Have confidence that you did the best you could.

APPENDIX A

☙ ☙ ☙

VBACs, Cesareans, and Infant Mortality Around the World

The infant mortality rate refers to the number of babies who die in their first year of life per one thousand births. Throughout most of the twentieth century, many developed nations have kept track of this rate, based mostly on information from birth certificates. Healthcare observers around the world give considerable importance to infant mortality, because small differences in this marker tell a great deal about other health-related aspects of a country, such as access to food, shelter, education, sanitation, and health care. Japan has the lowest infant mortality rate and, despite its high-density living conditions, ranks number one in many health indicators, including life expectancy for women. The United States is twenty-second on the infant mortality list, even though, per capita, it outspends each of the twenty-one countries ahead of it.

I sent requests to thirty countries, including the twenty-one nations with lower infant mortality rates than the United States. Most responded, though not all. I also received information from Argentina, Russia, and China, all of whose infant mortality rates are many times higher than those nations included on the charts that follow.

The first chart shows infant mortality, cesarean, and VBAC rates for all countries ahead of the United States on the list. The second chart shows only VBAC rates; it includes just the seven countries that I know of that currently track this statistic. In Chart #1, a box that says "Not available" indicates that the given country does not track the cesarean or the VBAC statistic. A blank space indicates that I received no data from that particular country.

Chart #1: Infant Mortality, Cesarean, and VBAC Rates

COUNTRY	INFANT MORTALITY RATE	CESAREAN RATE	VBAC RATE
1. Japan	4.2	11.2	Not available
2. Singapore	4.3	27.0	70.0 (after 1 cesarean)
3. Sweden	4.4	12.0	Not available
4. Finland	4.7	15.4	40.4
5. Hong Kong	4.8	Not available	Not available
6. Norway	5.2	12.5	54.1
7. Switzerland	5.5	Not available	Not available
8. Denmark	5.6		
9. Germany	5.6	17.0	Not available
10. Ireland	5.9		
11. Netherlands	5.9	9.2	Not available
12. Australia	5.9	17.5	Not available
13. Austria	6.1	12.4	Not available
14. France	6.1		
15. Canada	6.2	17.6	33.4
16. United Kingdom: England, Scotland, Wales, Northern Ireland	6.2	England, 15.0 Scotland, 15.9 Wales and Northern Ireland, not available	Not available 43.2
17. Italy	6.7	22.4	
18. New Zealand	7.2 (1993)		
19. Spain	7.2	17.7	Not available
20. Portugal	7.4	24.3	Not available
21. Belgium	7.6		
22. United States	8.0	20.8	35.5

Unless otherwise indicated, all statistics are for 1994–1995. The infant mortality rates are from "Annual Summary of Vital Statistics—1995," by Bernard Guyer, et al., *Pediatrics* 98(6), 1996, with the exception of the following countries, who sent me their information: Denmark, Germany, Hong Kong, and Portugal. The VBAC and cesarean rates were provided by multiple sources, which are cited below. All correspondence with statisticians in individual countries occurred between December 1996 and June 1997.

1. **Japan:** Kanegae, Yoko. Japanese Statistics and Information Department, Tokyo.
2. **Singapore:** Emmanuel, S. C. Epidemiology and Disease Control Department, Singapore.
3. **Sweden:** Johansson, Eva. Swedish Medical Birth Registry, Stockholm.
4. **Finland:** Gissler, Mika. Finnish Medical Birth Register, Helsinki.
5. **Hong Kong:** Yeung, Simon. Department of Health, Hong Kong.
6. **Norway:** Edland, Ole-Henrik. Medical Birth Registry of Norway, Bergen.
7. **Switzerland:** Wuest, Erwin. Swiss Federal Statistical Office, Bern.
8. **Denmark:** No response.
9. **Germany:** Hammer, K. J. Statistisches Bundesamt, Wiesbaden.
10. **Ireland:** No response.
11. **Netherlands:** Van Hussen, J. Statistics Netherlands, Voorburg.
12. **Australia:** Wood, Tony. Australian Bureau of Statistics, Sydney.
13. **Austria:** Langgassner, Jeannette. Austrian Central Statistical Office, Vienna.
14. **France:** No response.
15. **Canada:** Hagey, Janet. Statistics Canada, Ottawa.
    Millar, Wayne J., et al. "Declining Cesarean Section Rates: A Continuing Trend?" *Canadian Health Reports* 8(1), 1996.
16. **United Kingdom:** Health Committee. Public Expenditure on Health and Personal Social Services, London. Printed for the House of Commons, October 1996.
    Hamilton, Patricia. Northern Ireland Statistics & Research Agency, Belfast.
    Hollinsworth, Mark. Information and Statistics Division, Edinburgh.
17. **Italy:** "Italy Has Europe's Highest Cesarean Section Rate." *British Medical Journal* 310 (1995).
18. **New Zealand:** No response.
19. **Spain:** Arribas, Carmen. Oficina de Relaciones Internacionales, Madrid.
20. **Portugal:** Leal, Joao C. Farrajota. Instituto Nacional de Estatistica, Lisbon.
21. **Belgium:** No response.
22. **United States:** Clarke, Sally. National Center for Health Statistics, Hyattsville, Maryland.

Others who provided information include Julio A. Roca, Instituto Nacional de Estadistica y Censos, Buenos Aires; Xiaoyan Ren, International Statistical Information Center, Beijing; and A. Savinykh, Public Health Institute, Moscow.

Chart #2: International VBAC Rates

COUNTRY	VBAC RATE
1. Singapore	70.0 (after 1 cesarean only)
2. Israel	55.1 (1992)
3. Norway	54.1
4. Scotland	43.2
5. Finland	40.4
6. United States	35.5
7. Canada	33.4

The Israel rate is from 1992 and the Canada rate is from 1993. All others are from 1995.

Sources: Except for the statistics for Israel, the list of citations following Chart #1 ("Infant Mortality, Cesarean, and VBAC Rates") also includes the sources used for the statistics presented in Chart #2.

Israel: Mor-Yosef, S., et al. "The Israel Perinatal Census." *Asia Oceania Journal of Obstetrics and Gynaecology* (18)2, 1992.

Chart #3: International Cesarean Rates

COUNTRY	CESAREAN RATE
1. Netherlands	9.2
2. Japan	11.2
3. Sweden	12.0
4. Austria	12.4
5. Norway	12.5
6. England	15.0
7. Finland	15.4
8. Scotland	15.9
9. Germany	17.0
10. Australia	17.5
11. Canada	17.6
12. Spain	17.7
13. United States	20.8
14. Italy	22.4
15. Portugal	24.3
16. Singapore	27.0
17. Chile	36.0
18. Brazil	38.0 (public hospitals)
	75.0 (private clinics)

Sources: The statistics for the first 16 countries come from the list of citations following Chart #1 ("Infant Mortality, Cesarean, and VBAC Rates").

Chile: Odent, Michel. Letter to author, January 26, 1997.

Brazil: de Mello e Souza, Cecilia. "C-sections as Ideal Births: The Cultural Constructions of Beneficence and Patients' Rights in Brazil." *Cambridge Quarterly of Healthcare Ethics* 3, 1994.

APPENDIX B

❧ ❧ ❧

Resource Directory

For those of you lucky enough to have access to e-mail or the Internet, I've provided web sites and e-mail addresses when available. In fact, the Internet is a rich source of VBAC support and information. Only those organizations, however, which provide phone numbers and mailing addresses, as well as e-mail and Internet addresses, are included in this directory. To find Internet VBAC resources not listed here, put the acronym "VBAC" into one of the many Internet search engines.

Please keep in mind that names, addresses, and phone numbers (and often area codes) change frequently, particularly in the case of a volunteer organization. If you find that any of the numbers or addresses in this directory is incorrect by the time you need to use it, call the reference room of your library for updated information. Toll-free numbers are those with 1-800 or 1-888 prefixes.

If you are affiliated with an organization listed here and you know that it has moved, or if you know of a group that fits into one of the categories in this directory but is not listed, please notify me, Diana Korte, either c/o Harvard Common Press, 535 Albany Street, Boston, MA 02118 or by e-mail at DianaKorte@aol.com.

"SASE" means send a self-addressed, stamped, business-size envelope if you are requesting information. (Some listings for resources outside of the United States specify a C5-size envelope, which is the British business-size envelope.)

Contents

VBAC Resources

Birth After Cesarean Unlimited Possibilities (BACUP)
P.O. Box 4059
Kingston, ACT, Australia 2604
Internet home page: http://edsitewa.iinet.net.au/bacup
Since 1989 has provided encouragement, support, and information about VBAC through meetings, a bimonthly newsletter, and its book, *Birth After Cesarean: Unlimited Possibilities.*

Nancy Wainer Cohen
10 Great Plain Terrace
Needham, MA 02192
(617) 449-2490
e-mail: cmousse2@aol.com
Activist and VBAC counselor since 1972 who coined the term "VBAC." Teaches workshops nationwide on healing after traumatic births and other topics; is available for consultation by appointment. Both of her books, *Silent Knife* (1983) and *Open Season* (1991), can be ordered from her directly.

C/SEC, Inc. (Cesareans/Support, Education and Concern)
22 Forest Road
Framingham, MA 01701
(508) 877-8266
Since 1973 has served as a resource for publications, local support groups, and regional contacts for phone counseling about VBACs. Send SASE.

Valerie El Halta, co-director
The Birth Center
5460 Schaefer
Dearborn, MI 48126
(313) 582-9353

Direct-entry midwife for more than twenty years and has assisted at more than 2,500 births, including 200 VBACs, in which every posterior baby has been successfully turned. Has a 100 percent VBAC success rate. Copies of her complete article, "Posterior Labor—A Pain in the Back! Its Prevention and Cure" (1991), referred to in Chapter 3, are available. The article includes specific details for healthcare providers on turning a posterior baby in labor. Send $2.50 and SASE.

International Cesarean Awareness Network (ICAN)
1304 Kingsdale Avenue
Redondo Beach, CA 90278
phone: (310) 542-6400; fax: (310) 542-5368
e-mail: ICANinc@aol.com
Internet home page: http://www.childbirth.org/section/ICAN/html

Since 1982 has provided information on cesarean birth: referrals to VBAC-friendly doctors and midwives, support groups, network access, and a quarterly newsletter, *The Clarion*.

MotherWorks
Robin Elise Weiss
11707 Saratoga Woods Court
Louisville, KY 40299
e-mail: robin@childbirth.org
Internet home page: http://www.childbirth.org

Web site is one of the most comprehensive pregnancy and childbirth sites on the Internet. For readers who want a printed copy of "The VBAC Frequently Asked Questions" page, a periodically updated list of common VBAC questions and informative answers to them, send an SASE with two stamps.

Public Citizen Health Research Group
1600 20th Street, NW
Washington, DC 20009
(202) 588-1000 (publications)

Offers reports by state on hospitals' cesarean and VBAC rates for forty-one states. Each report costs $15; the last update was in 1997.

Lynn Baptisti Richards
3455 Moki Drive
Sedona, AZ 86336
(520) 282-9787
e-mail: lbrdam@sedona.com
Midwife for twenty years and VBAC counselor since 1978. Offers a spiritual and emotionally based counseling service. She is the author of *The Vaginal Birth After Cesarean Experience* (Bergin & Garvey, 1988). Her other two books, *VBAC and Cesarean Counseling: A Handbook for Midwives* (1990) and *The VBAC Experience* (1990), can be ordered from her directly.

VBAC Information & Support
Linda Howes
8 Wren Way
Farnborough, Hants
GU14 8SZ England
phone/fax: (01252) 543250
phone/pager: (0839) 612195 (use only if no answer at above number)
e-mail: Lynvbac@aol.com
Provides a newsletter, contacts in the United Kingdom and eighteen other countries, a comprehensive lending library of more than eighty titles, VBAC planning and postcesarean counseling, and extensive resources (available for a small fee). Calls are welcome between 9:30 A.M. and 9:00 P.M., seven days a week. SASE with C5-size envelope.

Other Birth Resources

BIRTH AND LABOR ASSISTANTS, DOULAS, LABOR COACHES

Academy of Certified Birth Educators and Labor Support Professionals
2001 East Prairie Circle, Suite 1
Olathe, KS 66502
phone: (800) 444-8223; fax: (913) 397-0933
Provides three-day certification program for childbirth educators and those training to be doulas in cities around the country.

Association of Labor Assistants and Childbirth Educators (ALACE)
P.O. Box 382724
Cambridge, MA 02238

phone: (617) 441-2500; fax: (617) 441-3167
e-mail: alacehq@aol.com
Internet home page: http://www.alace.org
Provides training for childbirth educators and labor assistants, consumer referrals, and publications, including *Special Delivery,* a quarterly magazine.

The Birth Institute
1126 Solano Avenue
Albany, CA 94706
phone: (510) 527-2121; fax: (510) 559-5518
Provides training for labor assistants, called "birth guides," through classes and workshops; offers other pregnancy and postpartum classes.

Doulas of North America (DONA)
1100 23rd Avenue East
Seattle, WA 98112
phone: (206) 324-5440
Internet home page: http://www.dona.com
Provides information about membership, training, and certification to anyone wishing to become a birth doula (labor support provider) and referrals to those looking for a doula to support them during their labor and birth. SASE preferred.

International Childbirth Education Association (ICEA)
P.O. Box 20048
Minneapolis, MN 55420
phone: (612) 854-8660; fax: (612) 854-8772
e-mail: info@icea.org
Internet home page: http://www.icea.org
Provides certification programs for childbirth educators, postnatal educators, and doulas; offers publications (mail-order book catalog, pamphlets, video, audio tapes, and teaching aids), workshops, and annual conference.

Seattle Midwifery School
2524 16th Avenue South, #300
Seattle, WA 98144
phone: (206) 322-8834; fax: (206) 328-2840
Provides midwifery education, labor support and postpartum doula training, and other continuing education and advocacy programs.

BIRTH CENTERS

National Association of Childbearing Centers (NACC)
3123 Gottchall Road
Perkiomenville, PA 18074
phone: (215) 234-8068; fax: (215) 234-8829
e-mail: birthctr@midwives.org
Collects and disseminates information on birth centers staffed by certified
nurse-midwives and physicians; holds annual meeting and regional workshops. Contact for list of birth centers in your area and guidelines on how to
select one. Send $1 for postage and handling.

Non-NACC Birth Centers
Some, but not all, staffed by direct-entry midwives. To locate non-NACC
birth centers, look in your yellow pages or local parenting magazines, contact the midwifery organizations listed elsewhere in this directory, or call
childbirth educators in your area.

BIRTH PUBLICATIONS

Birth Gazette
42, The Farm
Summertown, TN 38483
phone: (615) 964-2519
Quarterly magazine for midwives, physicians, childbirth educators, parents,
breastfeeding counselors, health planners, and legislators.

The Compleat Mother
P.O. Box 209
Minot, ND 58702
phone: (701) 852-2822 (in U.S.), (519) 327-8785 (in Canada)
fax: (519) 364-7036 (in Canada)
e-mail: zyoung@wcl.on.ca
Quarterly magazine of pregnancy, birth, and breastfeeding, with stories of
adoption lactation success, home waterbirth, and life without doctors.

Midwifery Today
P.O. Box 2672
Eugene, OR 97402

phone: (800) 743-0974 or (541) 344-1422
fax: (541) 344-1422
e-mail: midwifery@aol.com
Internet home page: http://members.aol.com/midwifery
Quarterly magazine for and by birth practitioners, childbirth educators, midwives, parents, doctors, and nurses.

Mothering magazine
P.O. Box 1690
Santa Fe, NM 87504
phone: (800) 984-8116 or (505) 984-8116
fax: (505) 986-8335
e-mail: mother@ni.net
Quarterly magazine that celebrates parenting, advocates the needs and rights of the child, and provides information on which parents can base informed choices.

CHILDBIRTH CLASSES

Academy of Certified Birth Educators
(see listing under "Birth and Labor Assistants, Doulas, and Labor Coaches")

ASPO/Lamaze
1200 19th Street, NW, Suite 300
Washington, DC 20036
phone: (800) 368-4404; fax: (202) 223-4579
e-mail: aspo@sba.com
Internet home page: http://www.lamaze-childbirth.com
Provides referrals to Lamaze educators, information on the Lamaze method, and a catalog of books, tapes, and related materials.

Association of Labor Assistants and Childbirth Educators (ALACE)
(see listing under "Birth and Labor Assistants, Doulas, and Labor Coaches")

Birth Works
P.O. Box 2045
Medford, NJ 08055
phone: (888) TO-BIRTH or (609) 953-9380
fax: (609) 953-9380

e-mail: birthwkscd@aol.com

Internet home page: http://members.aol.com/birthwkscd/bw.html
Provides childbirth education and teacher certification program designed to develop a woman's self-confidence, trust, and faith in her innate ability to give birth. Also offers regional workshops and newsletter. SASE with 55¢ stamp.

The Bradley Method® (formerly American Academy of Husband-Coached Childbirth)
    P.O. Box 5224
    Sherman Oaks, CA 91413
    phone: (800) 4-A-BIRTH or (818) 788-6662
    Internet home page: http://www.bradleybirth.com
Provides referrals to the Bradley Method® childbirth classes and sends free package of information.

Childbirth Without Pain Education Association
    20134 Snowden Street
    Detroit, MI 48235
    phone: (313) 341-3876
Provides Lamaze classes for expectant parents; teacher training and certification, monitrice training, and film programs. SASE.

International Childbirth Education Association
(see listing under "Birth and Labor Assistants, Doulas, and Labor Coaches")

Read Natural Childbirth Foundation
    P.O. Box 150956
    San Rafael, CA 94915
    phone: (415) 456-8462
Offers Grantly Dick-Read childbirth education program, labor support service, and video and book library.

CHILDBIRTH ORGANIZATIONS

Alliance for the Improvement of Maternity Services (AIMS)
    American Foundation for Maternal and Child Health (AFMCH)
    439 East 51st Street
    New York, NY 10022

phone: (212) 759-5510; fax: (212) 935-0191
e-mail: aims@comet.net
Internet home page: htpp://www.comet.net/aims
AIMS seeks to reduce birth injury and trauma in newborns and mothers through sharing of scientific and public information. AFMCH promotes unmedicated childbirth by sponsoring research seminars, publishing literature, and exerting pressures on national and state legislators and agencies.

NAPSAC International
Route 1, Box 646
Marble Hill, MO 63764
phone: (573) 238-2010; fax: (573) 238-2010
Promotes education about all childbirth alternatives with newsletter, books, and other publications, including the *NAPSAC Directory of Alternative Birth Services.*

CLAIMS CONSULTANTS

National Association of Claims Assistance Professionals
5329 South Main Street, #102
Downers Grove, IL 60515
phone: (630) 963-3500
Offers referrals to members who help consumers resolve disputes with insurance companies and hospital billing departments. NACAP has members in every state, with 2,000 members in the entire organization. Include $1 when requesting a referral.

MIDWIVES

American College of Nurse-Midwives (ACNM)
818 Connecticut Avenue, NW, Suite 900
Washington, DC 20006
phone: (888) MIDWIFE or (202) 728-9860; fax: (202) 728-9897
e-mail: info@acnm.org
Internet home page: http://www.midwife.org
Provides information regarding nurse-midwives around the country.

Association of Ontario Midwives
   562 Eglinton Avenue East, Suite 102
   Toronto, Ontario
   Canada M4P 1B9
   phone: (416) 481-2811; fax: (416) 481-7547
   e-mail: midwives@interlog.com
Provides referrals to midwives in Ontario.

California Association of Midwives
   P.O. Box 417854
   Sacramento, CA 95841
   phone: (800) 829-5791
Provides information on midwifery and referrals to California midwives.

Informed Homebirth/Informed Birth & Parenting (IH/IBP)
   P.O. Box 3675
   Ann Arbor, MI 48106
   phone: (313) 662-6857
Provides information about alternatives in birth and parenting, referrals to midwives, childbirth educators, and birth assistants; offers books, videos, and two annual conferences.

Midwives Alliance of North America (MANA)
   P.O. Box 175
   Newton, KS 67114
   e-mail: manainfo@aol.com
   Internet home page: http://www.mana.org
Promotes midwifery as a means of improving health care, encourages cooperation among midwives, and improves quality and availability of educational opportunities for midwives. Maintains a current list of midwifery organizations by state.

Seattle Midwifery School
(see listing under "Birth and Labor Assistants, Doulas, and Labor Coaches")

MOTHER-HELPERS

National Association of Postpartum Care Services (NAPCS)
11 Bronxville Road, Apartment 1C
Bronxville, NY 10708
phone: (800) 45-DOULA or (914) 793-8307
Provides referrals to consumers for postpartum doulas, certification of postpartum doulas, and accreditation of doula services. Lobbies government and insurance companies, hosts national conferences, and has a published cookbook.

VIDEOS

Injoy Productions
3970 Broadway, Suite B4
Boulder, CO 80304
phone: (800) 326-2082 or (303) 447-2082
fax: (303) 449-8788
Provides free catalog of birth and parenting educational videos, including *Birth Stories Video Library* (this includes more than fifteen birth stories, two of them VBACs), *Special Women: How a Labor Assistant Makes Birth Safer, More Satisfying, and Less Expensive,* and *Cesarean Births—Personal Stories and Preparation for the Unexpected Cesarean.*

✿ ✿ ✿

Bibliographic References
(by Chapter)

Introduction

History of VBACs and Cesareans

Flamm, Bruce L. "Once a Cesarean, Always a Controversy." *Obstetrics & Gynecology* 90(2), 1997.

Korte, Diana. *Every Woman's Body* (New York: Ballantine, 1994).

A Note on Gender

Awaakye, Barbara. Correspondence with information officer at the American College of Obstetricians and Gynecologists, Washington, DC, March 10, 1997.

VBAC Statistics

Clarke, Sally. Correspondence and conversations with healthcare statistician, National Center for Health Statistics, Hyattsville, MD, January and February 1997.

Chapter 1. Have a VBAC—Here's Why

Advantages for Babies Born by VBAC

Hansell, R. S., et al. "Vaginal Birth After Two or More Cesarean Sections: A Five-Year Experience." *Birth* 17(3), 1990.

Iffy, L., et al. "Rates of Cesarean Section and Perinatal Outcome. Perinatal Mortality." *Acta Obstetricia et Gynecologica Scandinavica* 73(3), 1994.

Myers, Stephen A., and Norbert Gleicher. "A Program to Lower Cesarean-Section Rates." *New England Journal of Medicine* 320(25), 1989.

O'Driscoll, K., et al. "Cesarean Section and Perinatal Outcome: Response from the House of Horne." *American Journal of Obstetrics and Gynecology* 158(3), 1988.

Sepkowitz, S. "Birth Weight—Specific Fetal Deaths and Neonatal Mortality and the Rising Cesarean Section Rate." *Journal of the Oklahoma State Medical Association* 85(5), 1992.

Shearer, Elizabeth L. "Cesarean Section: Medical Benefits and Costs." *Social Science and Medicine* 37(10), 1993.

Taylor, U., et al. "Rates of Caesarean Section and Neonatal Mortality." *Australian and New Zealand Journal of Obstetrics and Gynaecology* 32(3), 1992.

Better Apgar

Andersen, H. F., et al. "Neonatal Status in Relation to Incision Internals, Obstetric Factors, and Anesthesia at Cesarean Delivery." *American Journal of Perinatology* 4(4), 1987.

Annibale, D. J., et al. "Comparative Neonatal Morbidity of Abdominal and Vaginal Deliveries After Uncomplicated Pregnancies." *Archives of Pediatrics and Adolescent Medicine* 149(8), 1995.

Crawford, J. Selwyn, and Paul Davies. "Status of Neonates Delivered by Elective Caesarean Section." *British Journal of Anaesthesia* 54, 1982.

Birth Canal Hormones

Faxelius, G., et al. "Catecholamine Surge and Lung Function After Delivery." *Archives of Diseases in Childhood* 58(4), 1983.

Hagnevik, K., et al. "Establishment of Functional Residual Capacity in Infants Delivered Vaginally and by Elective Cesarean Section." *Early Human Development* 27(1–2), 1991.

Lagercrantz, Hugo, and Theodore A. Slotkin. "The 'Stress' of Being Born." *Scientific American,* April 1986.

Seidler, Frederic. Phone interview with catacholamine researcher, Duke University Medical School, Durham, NC, June 12, 1997.

Born on Time

Centers for Disease Control and Prevention/National Center for Health Statistics. "Advance Report of Final Natality Statistics, 1994." *Monthly Vital Statistics Report* 44(11), 1996.

Nathanielsz, Peter W. "The Timing of Birth." *American Scientist* November–December 1996.

Cesareans and VBACs Around the World

Howes, Linda. Correspondence via e-mail, February–March 1997.

Lidegaard, O., et al. "Technology Use, Cesarean Section Rates, and Perinatal Mortality at Danish Maternity Wards." *Acta Obstetricia et Gynecologica Scandinavica* 73(3), 1994.

(See information in Appendix A for all additional references.)

Early Contact and Breastfeeding

Chen, Yue. "Factors Associated with Artificial Feeding in Shanghai." *American Journal of Public Health* 82(2), 1992.

Ever-Hadani, P. "Breastfeeding in Israel: Maternal Factors Associated with Choice and Duration." *Journal of Epidemiology and Community Health* 48(3), 1994.

Ford, K., et al. "Who is Breast-Feeding? Implications of Associated Social and Biomedical Variables for Research on the Consequences of Methods of Infant Feeding." *American Journal of Clinical Nursing* 52, 1990.

Kearney, M. H., et al. "Cesarean Delivery and Breastfeeding Outcomes." *Birth* 17(2), 1990.

Mathur, G. P., et al. "Breastfeeding in Babies Delivered by Cesarean Section." *Indian Pediatrics* 30(11), 1993.

Newman, J. "Breastfeeding Problems Associated with the Early Introduction of Bottles and Pacifiers." *Journal of Human Lactation* 6(2), 1990.

Nylander, G., et al. "Unsupplemented Breastfeeding in the Maternity Ward. Positive Long-term Effects." *Acta Obstetricia et Gynecologica Scandinavica* 70(3), 1991.

Righard, L., and M. O. Alade. "Effect of Delivery Room Routines on Success of First Breast-Feed." *Lancet* 336, 1990.

Yamauchi, Y., and Itsuro Yamanouchi. "The Relationship Between Rooming-In/Not Rooming-In and Breast-Feeding Variables." *Acta Paediatricia Scandinavica* 79(11), 1990.

Healthy Lungs

Bryan, H., et al. "Perinatal Factors Associated with the Respiratory Distress Syndrome." *American Journal of Obstetrics and Gynecology* 162(2), 1990.

Chervenak, F. A., et al. "Current Perspectives on Iatrogenic Neonatal Respiratory Distress Syndrome." *Journal of Reproductive Medicine* 31(1), 1986.

Gale, Rena, et al. "Increased Neonatal Risk from the Use of General Anesthesia in Emergency Cesarean Section." *Journal of Reproductive Medicine* 27(11), 1982.

Hales, K. A., et al. "Influence of Labor and Route of Delivery on the

Frequency of Respiratory Morbidity in Term Neonates." *International Journal of Gynaecology and Obstetrics* 43(1), 1993.

Parilla, B. V., et al. "Iatrogenic Respiratory Distress Syndrome Following Elective Repeat Cesarean Delivery." *Obstetrics & Gynecology* 81(3), 1993.

Infant Mortality

Guyer, Bernard, et al. "Annual Summary of Vital Statistics—1995." *Pediatrics* 98(6), December 1996.

Kanegae, Yoko. Correspondence with healthcare statistician, Japanese Statistics and Information Department, Tokyo, January and February 1997.

Korte, Diana. "Infant Mortality: Lessons from Japan." *Mothering,* Winter 1992.

Notzon, Francis C. "International Differences in the Use of Obstetric Interventions." *Journal of the American Medical Association* 263(24), 1990.

Lower Risk for Infection

Bashore, R. A., et al. "A Comparison on the Morbidity of Midforceps and Cesarean Delivery." *American Journal of Obstetrics and Gynecology* 162(6), 1990.

Chang, P. L., and E. R. Newton. "Predictors of Antibiotic Prophylactic Failure in Post-Cesarean Endometritis." *Obstetrics & Gynecology* 80(1), 1992.

Cowan, R. K., et al. "Trial of Labor Following Cesarean Delivery." *Obstetrics & Gynecology* 83(6), 1994.

Eisenkop, Scott M., et al. "Urinary Tract Injury During Cesarean Section." *Obstetrics & Gynecology* 60(5), 1982.

Emmons, S. L., et al. "Development of Wound Infections Among Women Undergoing Cesarean Section." *Obstetrics & Gynecology* 72(4), 1988.

Eschenbach, D. A. "New Concepts of Obstetric and Gynecologic Infection." *Archives of Internal Medicine* 142(11), 1982.

Evans, L. C., and C. A. Combs. "Increased Maternal Morbidity After Cesarean Delivery Before 28 Weeks of Gestation." *International Journal of Gynaecology and Obstetrics* 40(3), 1993.

Flamm, Bruce L. "Once a Cesarean, Always a Controversy." *Obstetrics & Gynecology* 90(2), 1997.

Gonik, Bernard, et al. "Why Patients Fail Antibiotic Prophylaxis at Cesarean Delivery: Histologic Evidence for Incipient Infection." *Obstetrics & Gynecology* 79(2), 1992.

Hagglund, Leif, et al. "Risk Factors in Cesarean Section Infection." *Obstetrics & Gynecology* 62(2), 1983.

Hawrylyshyn, P. A., et al. "Short-Term Antibiotic Prophylaxis in High-Risk Patients Following Cesarean Section." *American Journal of Obstetrics and Gynecology* 145(3), 1983.

Hemminki, E. "Long-Term Maternal Health Effects of Caesarean Section." *Journal of Epidemiology and Community Health* 45(1), 1991.

Henderson, E., and E. J. Love. "Incidence of Hospital-Acquired Infections Associated with Caesarean Section." *Journal of Hospital Infection* 29(4), 1995.

Hillan, E. M. "Postoperative Morbidity Following Caesarean Delivery." *Journal of Advanced Nursing* 22(6), 1995.

Magann, E. F., et al. "Infections, Morbidity, Operative Blood Loss, and Length of the Operative Procedure After Cesarean Delivery by Method of Placental Removal and Site of Uterine Repair." *Journal of American College of Surgeons* 181(6), 1995.

Magee, K. P., et al. "Endometritis After Cesarean: The Effect of Age." *American Journal of Perinatology* 11(1), 1994.

Martens, M. G., et al. "Development of Wound Infection or Separation After Cesarean Delivery. Prospective Evaluation of 2,431 Cases." *Journal of Reproductive Medicine* 40(3), 1995.

McMahon, M. J., et al. "Comparison of Trial of Labor with an Elective Second Cesarean Section." *New England Journal of Medicine* 335, 1996.

Middleton, J. R., et al. "Post-Cesarean Section Endometritis: Causative Organisms and Risk Factors." *American Journal of Obstetrics and Gynecology* 137(1), 1980.

Miller, P. J., et al. "The Relationship Between Surgeon Experience and Endometritis After Cesarean Section." *Surgery, Gynecology and Obstetrics* 165(6), 1987.

Pelle, H., et al. "Wound Infection After Cesarean Section." *Infection Control* 7(9), 1986.

Perlow, J. H., and M. A. Morgan. "Massive Maternal Obesity and Peri-operative Cesarean Morbidity." *American Journal of Obstetrics and Gynecology* 170(2), 1994.

Rosen, M. G., et al. "Vaginal Birth After Cesarean: A Meta-Analysis of Morbidity and Mortality." *Obstetrics & Gynecology* 77(3), 1991.

Stafford, Randall S. "The Cesarean Section Rate." *Journal of the American Medical Association* 264(8), 1990.

Thompson, J. R., et al. "Estimating the Infection Rate in Mothers Following Caesarean Section." *Journal of Hospital Infection* 10(2), 1987.

Watts, D. H., et al. "Bacterial Vaginosis as a Risk Factor for Post-Cesarean

Endometritis." *Obstetrics & Gynecology* 75(1), 1990.

Yancey, M. K., et al. "The Frequency of Glove Contamination During Cesarean Delivery." *Obstetrics & Gynecology* 83(4), 1994.

Younis, M. N., et al. "The Febrile Morbidity Score as a Predictor of Febrile Morbidity Following Cesarean Section." *International Journal of Gynaecology and Obstetrics* 35(3), 1991.

Maternal Deaths

Atrash, H. K., et al. "Maternal and Perinatal Mortality." *Current Opinion in Obstetrics and Gynecology* 4(1), 1992.

"Cesarean Section." Medical Data Exchange (http://www.thriveonline.com), 1996.

Enkin, Murray, et al. "Labour and Delivery After Previous Caesarean Section," in Murray Enkin et al, eds., *A Guide to Effective Care in Pregnancy & Childbirth* (Oxford, England: Oxford University Press, 1995).

Kochanek, Kenneth, and Bettie L. Hudson. "Advance Report of Final Mortality Statistics, 1992." *Monthly Vital Statistics Report* 43(6), 1994.

Leary, Warren E. "Study Shows Deaths in Pregnancy Are Underreported." *New York Times,* July 31, 1996.

"Mortality Patterns—United States, 1993." *Morbidity and Mortality Weekly Report* 45(8), 1996.

Mukherji, J., and J. C. Samaddar. "How Safe Is Caesarean Section?" *Journal of Obstetrics and Gynaecology* 21, 1995.

Petitti, Diana B., et al. "In-hospital Maternal Mortality in the United States: Time Trends and Relation to Method of Delivery." *Obstetrics & Gynecology* 59(1), 1982.

No Cesarean Depression

Affonso, Dyanne, and Jaynelle F. Stichler. "Cesarean Birth—Women's Reactions." *American Journal of Nursing,* March 1980.

Boyce, P. M., et al. "Increased Risk of Postnatal Depression After Emergency Caesarean Section." *Medical Journal of Australia* 157(3), 1992.

Cranley, Mecca S., et al. "Women's Perception of Vaginal and Cesarean Deliveries." *Nursing Research* 32(1), 1983.

Dimitrovsky, L., et al. "Depression During and Following Pregnancy: Quality of Family Relationships." *Journal of Psychology* 121(3), 1987.

Fawcett, Jacqueline. "Needs of Cesarean Birth Parents." *Journal of Obstetrical & Gynecological Nursing,* September/October 1981.

Fergusson, D. M., et al. "Relationship of Family Life Events, Maternal Depression, and Childrearing Problems." *Pediatrics* 73(6), 1984.

Goldbeck-Wood, Sandra. "Post-Traumatic Stress Disorder May Follow Childbirth." *British Medical Journal* 313, 1996.

Gottlieb, S. E. "Effects of Unanticipated Cesarean Section on Mothers, Infants, and Their Interaction in the First Month of Life." *Journal of Development and Behavior in Pediatrics* 7(3), 1986.

Hillan, E. M. "Short-Term Morbidity Associated with Cesarean Delivery." *Birth* 19(4), 1992.

Knight, R. G. "The Relationship Between Expectations of Pregnancy and Birth, and Transient Depression in the Immediate Postpartum Period." *Journal of Psychosomatic Research* 31(3), 1987.

Korte, Diana. *Every Woman's Body* (New York: Ballantine, 1994).

Kumar, R. "A Prospective Study of Emotional Disorders in Childbearing Women." *British Journal of Psychiatry* 144 (1984).

Lipson, Juliene G. "Cesarean Support Groups: Mutual Help and Education." *Women & Health* 6(3/4), 1987.

Lipson, Juliene G., et al. "Psychological Integration of the Cesarean Birth Experience." *American Journal of Orthopsychiatry* 50(4), 1980.

Richardson, Peggy. "The Body Boundary Experience of Women in Labor: A Framework for Care." *Maternal Child Nursing Journal* 13(2), 1984.

Sandelowski, M. "Cesarean Birth Outside the Natural Childbirth Culture." *Research in Nursing and Health* 9(2), 1986.

Sargent, Carolyn. "Surgical Birth: Interpretations of Cesarean Delivery Among Private Hospital Patients and Nursing Staff." *Social Science and Medicine* 25(12), 1987.

Stern, G. "Multi-Disciplinary Perspectives on Post-Partum Depression: An Anthropological Critique." *Social Science and Medicine* 17(15), 1983.

Stichler, Jaynelle F., and Dyanne D. Affonso. "Cesarean Birth." *American Journal of Nursing*, March 1980.

Tilden, V., and J. Lipson. "Cesarean Childbirth. Variables Affecting Psychological Impact." *Western Journal of Nursing Research* 3, 1981.

Trowell, Judith. "Possible Effects of Emergency Caesarian Section on the Mother-Child Relationship." *Early Human Development* 7 (1982).

Trowell, Judith Ann. "Emergency Caesarian Section: A Research Study of the Mother/Child Relationship of a Group of Women Admitted Expecting a Normal Vaginal Delivery." *Child Abuse and Neglect* 7, 1983.

Tulman, L. J. "Initial Handling of Newborns by Vaginally and Cesarean-Delivered Mothers." *Nursing Research* 35(5), 1986.

Placenta Previa and Placenta Accreta

Chazotte, C., and W. R. Cohen. "Catastrophic Complications of Previous Cesarean Section." *American Journal of Obstetrics and Gynecology* 163(3), 1990.

Cibils, Luis A. "Breech Presentation," in Bruce L. Flamm and Edward J. Quilligan, eds., *Cesarean Section: Guidelines for Appropriate Utilization* (New York: Springer-Verlag, 1995).

Clark, S. L., et al. "Placenta Previa/Accreta and Prior Cesarean Section." *Obstetrics & Gynecology* 66(1), 1985.

Finberg, H. J., and J. W. Williams. "Placenta Accreta: Prospective Sonographic Diagnosis in Patients with Placenta Previa and Prior Cesarean Section." *Journal of Ultrasound in Medicine* 11(7), 1992.

Hershkowitz, R., et al. "One or Multiple Previous Cesarean Sections Are Associated with Similar Increased Frequency of Placenta Previa." *European Journal of Obstetrics, Gynecology, & Reproductive Biology* 62(2), 1995.

Manyonda, I. T., and T. R. Varma. "Massive Obstetric Hemorrhage Due to Placenta Previa/Accreta with Prior Cesarean Section." *International Journal of Gynaecology and Obstetrics* 34(2), 1991.

Singh, P. M., et al. "Placenta Previa and Previous Cesarean Section." *Acta Obstetricia et Gynecologica Scandinavica* 60, 1981.

Stanco, L. M., et al. "Emergency Peripartum Hysterectomy and Associated Risk Factors." *American Journal of Obstetrics and Gynecology* 168(3, part 1), 1993.

Taylor, V. M., et al. "Placenta Previa and Prior Cesarean Delivery: How Strong Is the Association?" *Obstetrics & Gynecology* 84(1), 1994.

To, W. W., and W. C. Leung. "Placenta Previa and Previous Cesarean Section." *International Journal of Gynaecology and Obstetrics* 51(1), 1995.

VBAC Recovery

Roan, Shari. "The Fourth Trimester: Think It Takes Only Six Weeks to Bounce Back from Childbirth?" *Los Angeles Times*, May 24, 1994.

Tulman, L. J., and Jacqueline Fawcett. "Recovery from Childbirth: Looking Back 6 Months After Delivery." *Health Care of Women International* 12(3), 1991.

Tulman, L. J., and Jacqueline Fawcett. "Return of Functional Ability After Childbirth." *Nursing Research* 37(2), 1988.

VBAC Safety

The American Academy of Family Physicians Task Force on Clinical Policies for Patient Care. "Trial of Labor vs. Elective Repeat Cesarean Section." *American Family Physician* November 1, 1995.

American Academy of Pediatrics and American College of Obstetricians and Gynecologists. *Guidelines for Perinatal Care*, 3rd ed. (Washington, DC: American Academy of Pediatrics, 1992).

American College of Obstetricians and Gynecologists. "ACOG Practice Patterns: Vaginal Delivery After Previous Cesarean Birth." Number 1, August 1995.

Chapter 2. Overcome Your Fears of Having a VBAC

Effects of Sexual Abuse on Labor

Bachmann, Gloria A., et al. "Childhood Sexual Abuse and the Consequences in Adult Women." *Obstetrics & Gynecology* 71(4), 1988.

Courtois, Christine, and Clair Courtois Riley. "Pregnancy and Childbirth as Triggers for Abuse Memories: Implications for Care." *Birth* 19(4), 1992.

Holz, Karen A. "A Practical Approach to Clients Who Are Survivors of Childhood Sexual Abuse." *Journal of Nurse-Midwifery* 39(1), 1994.

National Center on Child Abuse and Neglect. *Study on National Incidence and Prevalence of Child Abuse and Neglect* (Washington, DC: U.S. Department of Health and Human Services, 1988).

Rhodes, Naomi, and Sally Hutchinson. "Labor Experiences of Childhood Sexual Abuse Survivors." *Birth* 21(4), 1994.

Rose, Anna. "Effects of Childhood Sexual Abuse on Childbirth: One Woman's Story." *Birth* 19(4), 1992.

Simkin, Penny. "Memories That Really Matter." *Childbirth Instructor* Winter 1994.

Simkin, Penny. "Overcoming the Legacy of Childhood Sexual Abuse: The Role of Caregivers and Childbirth Educators." *Birth* 19(4), 1992.

Van Derbur, Marilyn. Correspondence with former Miss America, incest survivor, and co-founder of "One Voice," Denver, CO, February and March 1997.

Uterine Scars and Risk for Rupture

American College of Obstetricians and Gynecologists. "ACOG Practice Patterns: Vaginal Delivery After Previous Cesarean Birth." Number 1, August 1995.

American College of Obstetricians and Gynecologists. "Vaginal Delivery After Previous Cesarean Birth." Number 1, August 1995.

Arbab, F., et al. "Uterine Rupture in First or Second Trimester of Pregnancy After In-Vitro Fertilization and Embryo Transfer." *Human Reproduction* 11(5), 1996.

Asakura, H., and S. A. Myers. "More Than One Previous Cesarean Delivery: A 5-Year Experience with 435 Patients." *Obstetrics & Gynecology* 85(6), 1995.

Chattopadhyay, S. K., et al. "Planned Vaginal Delivery After Two Previous Caesarean Sections." *British Journal of Obstetrics and Gynaecology* 101(6), 1994.

Cowan, Robert K., et al. "Trial of Labor Following Cesarean Delivery." *Obstetrics & Gynecology* 83(6), 1994.

Davies, J. A., and J. A. Spencer. "Trial of Scar." *British Journal of Hospital Medicine* 40(5), 1988.

Devoe, L. D., et al. "The Prediction of 'Controlled' Uterine Rupture by the Use of Intrauterine Pressure Catheters." *Obstetrics & Gynecology* 80(4), 1992.

Dibbs, K. I., et al. "Spontaneous Uterine Rupture and Hemoperitoneum in the First Trimester." *American Journal of Perinatology* 12(6), 1995.

Enkin, Murray, et al. "Labour and Delivery After Previous Caesarean Section," in *A Guide to Effective Care in Pregnancy & Childbirth*, in Murray Enkin et al, eds. (Oxford, England: Oxford University Press, 1995).

Farmer, R. M., et al. "Uterine Rupture During Trial of Labor After Previous Section." *American Journal of Obstetrics and Gynecology* 165(4, part 1) 1991.

Fedorkow, D. M., et al. "Ruptured Uterus in Pregnancy: A Canadian Hospital's Experience." *Canadian Medical Association Journal* 127(1), 1987.

Flamm, Bruce L. "Once a Cesarean, Always a Controversy." *Obstetrics & Gynecology* 90(2), 1997.

Flamm, Bruce L. "Vaginal Birth After Cesarean Section," in Bruce L. Flamm and Edward J. Quilligan, eds., *Cesarean Section: Guidelines for Appropriate Utilization* (New York: Springer-Verlag, 1995).

Friedmann, W., et al. "Uterine Rupture After Laparoscopic Myomectomy." *Acta Obstetricia et Gynecologica Scandinavica* 75(7), 1996.

Granovsky-Grisaru, S., et al. "The Management of Labor in Women with More Than One Uterine Scar: Is a Repeat Cesarean Section Really the Only 'Safe' Option?" *Journal of Perinatal Medicine* 22(1), 1994.

Haq, C. L. "Vaginal Birth After Cesarean Delivery." *American Family Physician* 37(6), 1988.

Krishnamurthy, S., et al. "The Role of Postnatal X-Ray Pelvimetry After

Caesarean Section in the Management of Subsequent Delivery." *British Journal of Obstetrics and Gynaecology* 98(7), 1991.

Lavin, J. P., et al. "Vaginal Delivery in Patients with a Prior Cesarean Section." *Obstetrics & Gynecology* 59(2), 1982.

Leung, Anna S., et al. "Risk Factors Associated with Uterine Rupture During Trial of Labor After Cesarean Delivery: A Case Control Study." *American Journal of Obstetrics and Gynecology* 168(6), 1993.

Martin, J. N., et al. "Vaginal Birth After Cesarean Section: The Demise of Routine Repeat Abdominal Delivery." *Obstetrical and Gynecological Clinics of North America* 15(4), 1988.

Maymon, R., et al. "Third-Trimester Uterine Rupture After Prostaglandin E2 for Labor Induction." *Journal of Reproductive Medicine* 37(21), 1992.

McMahon, Michael J., et al. "Comparison of a Trial of Labor with an Elective Second Cesarean Section." *New England Journal of Medicine* 335(10), 1996.

Miller, David A. "Vaginal Birth After Cesarean: A 10-Year Experience." *Obstetrics & Gynecology* 84(2), August 1994.

Miller, D. A., et al. "Vaginal Birth After Cesarean Section in Twin Gestation." *American Journal of Obstetrics and Gynecology* 175(1), 1996.

Naef, R. W., III, et al. "Trial of Labor After Cesarean Delivery with a Lower-Segment, Vertical Uterine Incision: Is It Safe?" *American Journal of Obstetrics and Gynecology* 172(6), 1995.

Paul, Richard. "Toward Fewer Cesarean Sections—The Role of a Trial Labor." *New England Journal of Medicine* 335(10), 1996.

Peaceman, Alan M., and John J. Sciarra. "Encouraging Trials of Labour for Patients with Previous Caesarean Birth." *Lancet* 347, 1996.

Pridjian, G. "Labor After Prior Cesarean Section." *Clinical Obstetrics and Gynecology* 35(3), 1992.

Rose, Sue. Interview with certified nurse-midwife on staff at Newton-Wellesley Hospital and The Birth Place at Wellesley, Wellesley, MA, March 6, 1997.

Rozenberg, P., et al. "Ultrasonographic Measurement of Lower Uterine Segment to Assess Risk of Defects of Scarred Uterus." *Lancet* 347, 1996.

Stalnaker, B. L., et al. "Characteristics of Sucessful Claims for Payment by the Florida Neurologic Injury Compensation Association Fund." *American Journal of Obstetrics and Gynecology* 177(2), 1997.

Sweeten, K. M., et al. "Spontaneous Rupture of the Unscarred Uterus." *American Journal of Obstetrics and Gynecology* 172(6), 1995.

Women Who Want Elective Repeat Cesareans

Abitbol, M. Maurice., et al. "Vaginal Birth After Cesarean Section: The Patient's Point of View." *American Family Physician* 47(1), 1993.

Atiba, E. O., et al. "Patients' Expectation and Caesarean Section Rate." *Lancet* 341 (1993).

Bickell, N. A., et al. "Effect of External Peer Review on Cesarean Delivery Rates: A Statewide Program." *Obstetrics & Gynecology* 87(5, part 1), 1996.

Cepicky, P., et al. "When Is It Possible to Meet the Wish of a Woman to Terminate Her Labour by Caesarean Section?" *European Journal of Obstetrics, Gynecology, & Reproductive Biology* 38(2), 1991.

Chapman, S. J., et al. "One- Versus Two-Layer Closure of a Low Transverse Cesarean: The Next Pregnancy." *Obstetrics & Gynecology* 89(1), 1997.

Davies, G. A., et al. "Vaginal Birth After Cesarean: Physicians' Perceptions and Practice." *Journal of Reproductive Medicine* 41(7), 1996.

Fawcett, J., et al. "Responses to Vaginal Birth After Cesarean Section." *Journal of Obstetric, Gynecologic, and Neonatal Nursing* 23(3), 1994.

Flamm, Bruce L. "The Patient Who Demands Cesarean Delivery," in Bruce L. Flamm and Edward J. Quilligan, eds., *Cesarean Section: Guidelines for Appropriate Utilization* (New York: Springer-Verlag, 1995).

Flamm, Bruce L. "Vaginal Birth After Cesarean Section," in Bruce L. Flamm and Edward J. Quilligan, eds., *Cesarean Section: Guidelines for Appropriate Utilization* (New York: Springer-Verlag, 1995).

Hanley, M. L., et al. "Analysis of Repeat Cesarean Delivery Indications: Implications of Heterogeneity." *American Journal of Obstetrics and Gynecology* 175(4, part 1), 1996.

Huggins, George R., and Asha Rijhsinghani-Bhatia. "Obstetrics and Gynecology." *Journal of the American Medical Association* 263(19), 1990.

Joseph, Gerald F., Jr., et al. "Vaginal Birth After Cesarean Section: The Impact of Patient Resistance to a Trial of Labor." *American Journal of Obstetrics and Gynecology* 164(6), 1991.

Kirk, E. Paul, et al. "Vaginal Birth After Cesarean or Repeat Cesarean Section: Medical Risks or Social Realities?" *American Journal of Obstetrics and Gynecology* 162(6), 1990.

Kline, J., and F. Arias. "Analysis of Factors Determining the Selection of Repeated Cesarean Section or Trial of Labor in Patients with Histories of Prior Cesarean Delivery." *Journal of Reproductive Medicine* 38(4), 1993.

McClain, Carol S. "The Making of a Medical Tradition: Vaginal Birth After Cesarean." *Social Science and Medicine* 31(2), 1990.

McClain, Carol S. "Patient Decision Making: The Case of Delivery Method After a Previous Cesarean Section." *Culture, Medicine, and Psychiatry* 11(4), 1987.

McClain, Carol S. "Why Women Choose Trial of Labor or Repeat Cesarean Section." *Journal of Family Practice* 14(3), 1985.

Miller, E. S., et al. "Vaginal Birth After Cesarean: A 5-Year Experience in a Family Practice Residency Program." *Journal of the American Board of Family Practice* 8(5), 1995.

"NEWS: The 1992 Cesarean Section Rate in the United States." *Birth* 12(2), 1994.

Norman, P., et al. "Elective Repeat Cesarean Sections: How Many Could Be Vaginal Births?" *Canadian Medical Association Journal* 149(4), 1993.

Oleske, D. M., et al. "Information Dissemination and the Cesarean Birth Rate. The Illinois Experience." *International Journal of Technology Assessment and Health Care* 8(4), 1992.

Roberts, R. G., et al. "Trial of Labor or Repeated Cesarean Section: The Woman's Choice." *Archives of Family Medicine* 6(2), 1997.

Ryding, E. L. "Investigation of 33 Women Who Demanded a Cesarean Section for Personal Reasons." *Acta Obstetricia et Gynecologica Scandinavica* 72(4), 1993.

Signorelli, C., et al. "Risk Factors for Caesarean Section in Italy: Results of a Multicentre Study." *Public Health* (England) 109(3), 1995.

Sperkling, L. S., et al. "Indications for Caesarean Section in Singleton Pregnancies in Two Danish Counties with Different Cesarean Section Rates." *Acta Obstetricia et Gynecologica Scandinavica* 73(2), 1994.

Vermont Program for Quality in Health Care, Inc. *Vermont Health Care Quality Report* (Montpelier, VT, 1996).

Chapter 3. Plan a Successful VBAC

Cesarean Malpractice Claims

American College of Obstetricians and Gynecologists. "Vaginal Birth After Cesarean Section: Report of a 1990 Survey of ACOG's Membership," August 28, 1990.

Eat Well

Balch, James F., and Phyllis A. Balch. *Prescription for Nutritional Healing*, 2nd ed. (Garden City Park, NY: Avery Publishing Group, 1996).

Brewer, Thomas H. *Metabolic Toxemia of Late Pregnancy: A Disease of Malnutrition* (New Canaan, CT: Keats Publishing, 1982).

National Academy of Sciences, Institute of Medicine. *Nutrition During Pregnancy. Part I: Weight Gain* (Washington, DC: National Academy Press, 1990).

Parker, J. D., and B. Abrams. "Prenatal Weight Gain Advice: An Examination of the Recent Prenatal Weight Gain Recommendations of the Institute of Medicine." *Obstetrics & Gynecology* 79(5, part 1), 1992.

Taffel, Selma, et al. "Medical Advice on Maternal Weight Gain and Actual Weight Gain." *Annals of the New York Academy of Sciences* 678, 1993.

Exercise Regularly

Artal, Raul, et al. "A Comparison of Cardiopulmonary Adaptations to Exercise in Pregnancy at Sea Level and Altitude." *American Journal of Obstetrics and Gynecology* 172(4, part 1), 1995.

Bell, R. J., et al. "The Effect of Vigorous Exercise During Pregnancy on Birth-Weight." *Australian and New Zealand Journal of Obstetrics and Gynaecology* 35(1), 1995.

Clapp, J. F., III. "The Course of Labor After Endurance Exercise During Pregnancy." *American Journal of Obstetrics and Gynecology* 163(6, part 1), 1990.

Clapp, J. F., III. "Effect of Recreational Exercise on Pregnancy Weight Gain and Subcutaneous Fat Deposition." *Medicine, Science, and Sports Exercise* 27(2), 1995.

Clapp, J. F., III. "Fetal Heart Rate Response to Running in Midpregnancy and Late Pregnancy." *American Journal of Obstetrics and Gynecology* 153(3), 1985.

Hatch, Maureen C., et al. "Maternal Exercise During Pregnancy, Physical Fitness, and Fetal Growth." *American Journal of Epidemiology* 137(10), 1993.

Horns, P. N., et al. "Pregnancy Outcomes Among Active and Sedentary Primiparous Women." *Journal of Obstetric, Gynecologic, and Neonatal Nursing* 25(1), 1996.

Koniak-Griffin, D. "Aerobic Exercise, Psychological Well-Being, and Physical Discomforts During Adolescent Pregnancy." *Research in Nursing & Health* 17(4), 1994.

Maring-Klug, R. "Reducing Low Back Pain During Pregnancy." *Nurse Practitioner* 7(10), 1982.

Sternfeld, B., et al. "Exercise During Pregnancy and Pregnancy Outcomes." *Medicine, Science, and Sports Exercise* 27(5), 1995.

Wallace, Arlene M., et al. "Aerobic Exercise, Maternal Self-Esteem, and Physical Discomforts During Pregnancy." *Journal of Nurse-Midwifery* 31(6), 1986.

Wolfe, L. A., and M. F. Mottola. "Aerobic Exercise in Pregnancy: An Update." *Canadian Journal of Applied Physiology* 18(2), 1993.

Failure of Ultrasound to Accurately Estimate Fetal Size

Adair, C. D., et al. "Labor Induction in Patients with Previous Cesarean Section." *American Journal of Perinatology* 12(6), 1995.

American College of Obstetricians and Gynecologists. "Fetal Macrosomia." *ACOG Technical Bulletin* 159 (September 1991).

Chauhan, S. P., et al. "Intrapartum Detection of a Macrosomic Fetus: Clinical Versus 8 Sonographic Models." *Australian and New Zealand Journal of Obstetrics and Gynecology* 35(3), 1995.

Chauhan, S. P., et al. "Parous Patients' Estimate of Birth Weight in Postterm Pregnancy." *Journal of Perinatology* 15(3), 1995.

Combs, C. A., et al. "Elective Induction Versus Spontaneous Labor After Sonographic Diagnosis of Fetal Macrosomia." *Obstetrics & Gynecology* 81(4), 1993.

Friesen, C. D., et al. "Influence of Spontaneous or Induced Labor on Delivering the Macrosomic Fetus." *American Journal of Perinatology* 12(1), 1995.

Hannah, M. E., et al. "Postterm Pregnancy: Putting the Merits of a Policy of Induction of Labor into Perspective." *Birth* 23(1), 1996.

Hedriana, H. L., and T. R. Moore. "A Comparison of Single Versus Multiple Growth Ultrasonographic Examinations in Predicting Birth Weight." *American Journal of Obstetrics and Gynecology* 170(6), 1994.

National Center for Health Statistics. "Work Table W-22A: Percent Distribution of Live Births by Period of Gestation, Race of Mother, and Live Birth Order—Total of 50 Reporting States and the District of Columbia, 1990," 1992.

Sandmire, H. F. "Whither Ultrasonic Prediction of Fetal Macrosomia?" *Obstetrics & Gynecology* 82(5), 1993.

Turner, M. J., et al. "The Influence of Birth Weight on Labor in Nulliparas." *Obstetrics & Gynecology* 76(2), 1990.

Weeks, J. W., et al. "Fetal Macrosomia: Does Antenatal Prediction Affect Delivery Route and Birth Outcome?" *American Journal of Obstetrics and Gynecology* 173(4), 1995.

Genital Herpes and Cesareans

American College of Obstetricians and Gynecologists. "Perinatal Herpes Simplex Virus Infections." *ACOG Technical Bulletin* 122 (November 1988).

Hensleigh, Paul A., et al. "Genital Herpes During Pregnancy: Inability to Distinguish Primary and Recurrent Infections Clinically." *Obstetrics & Gynecology* 89(6), 1997.

Overall, J. C., Jr. "Herpes Simplex Virus Infection of the Fetus and Newborn." *Pediatric Annual* 23(3), 1994.

Randolph, A. G., et al. "Cesarean Delivery for Women Presenting with Genital Herpes Lesions: Efficacy, Risks, and Costs." *Journal of the American Medical Association* 270(1), 1993.

Roberts, S. W., et al. "Genital Herpes During Pregnancy: No Lesions, No Cesarean." *Obstetrics & Gynecology* 85(2), 1995.

Scott, L. L., et al. "Acyclovir Suppression to Prevent Cesarean Delivery After First-Episode Genital Herpes." *Obstetrics & Gynecology* 87(1), 1996.

Predicting VBAC Success

Asakura, H., and S. A. Myers. "More Than One Previous Cesarean Delivery: A 5-Year Experience with 435 Patients." *Obstetrics & Gynecology* 85(6), 1995.

Cowan, Robert K., et al. "Trial of Labor Following Cesarean Delivery." *Obstetrics & Gynecology* 83(6), 1994.

Duff, P., et al. "Outcome of Trial of Labor in Patients with a Single Previous Low Transverse Cesarean Section for Dystocia." *Obstetrics & Gynecology* 71(3, part 1), 1988.

Hansell, R. S., et al. "Vaginal Birth After Two or More Cesarean Sections: A Five-Year Experience." *Birth* 17(3), 1990.

Iffy, L., et al. "Rates of Cesarean Section and Perinatal Outcome: Perinatal Mortality." *Acta Obstetricia et Gynecologica Scandinavica* 73(3), 1994.

Jakobi, Peter, et al. "Evaluation of Prognostic Factors for Vaginal Delivery After Cesarean Section." *Journal of Reproductive Medicine* 38(9), 1993.

King, D. E., and K. Lahiri. "Socioeconomic Factors and the Odds of Vaginal Birth After Cesarean Delivery." *Journal of the American Medical Association* 272(7), 1994.

Learman, L. A., et al. "Predictors of Repeat Cesarean Delivery After Trial of Labor: Do Any Exist?" *Journal of the American College of Surgeons* 182(3), 1996.

Martin, J. N., et al. "Vaginal Birth After Cesarean Section: The Demise of Routine Repeat Abdominal Delivery." *Obstetrical and Gynecological Clinics of*

North America 15(4), 1988.

McMahon, Michael J., et al. "Comparison of a Trial of Labor with an Elective Second Cesarean Section." *New England Journal of Medicine* 335(10), 1996.

Naef, R. W., III, et al. "Trial of Labor After Cesarean Delivery with a Lower-Segment, Vertical Uterine Incision: Is It Safe?" *American Journal of Obstetrics and Gynecology* 172(6), 1995.

Pickhardt, M. G., et al. "Vaginal Birth After Cesarean Delivery: Are There Useful and Valid Predictors of Success or Failure?" *American Journal of Obstetrics and Gynecology* 166(6, part 1), 1992.

Rosen, M. G., and J. C. Dickinson. "Vaginal Birth After Cesarean: A Meta-Analysis of Indicators for Success." *Obstetrics & Gynecology* 76(5, part 1), 1990.

Weinstein, D., et al. "Predictive Score for Vaginal Birth After Cesarean Section." *American Journal of Obstetrics and Gynecology* 174(1, part 1), 1996.

Reasons for Cesareans, Including Non-Medical Reasons

Anderson, G. M., et al. "Explaining Variations in Cesarean Section Rates: Patients, Facilities or Policies?" *Canadian Medical Association Journal* 132, 1985.

Berkowitz, Gertrud S., et al. "Effect of Physician Characteristics on the Cesarean Birth Rate." *American Journal of Obstetrics and Gynecology* 161, 1989.

Brodsky, Archie. "Prophylactic Cesarean Section at Term." *New England Journal of Medicine* 313(12), 1985.

Burns, L. R., et al. "The Effect of Physician Factors on the Cesarean Section Decision." *Medical Care* 33(4), 1995.

Clarke, Sally, and Selma Taffel. "Changes in Cesarean Delivery in the United States, 1988 and 1993." *Birth* 22(2), 1995.

Enkin, Murray W., and Walter J. Hannah. "Do Practice Guidelines Guide Practice?" *New England Journal of Medicine* 322(25), 1990.

Friedman, Emanuel A. "The Obstetrician's Dilemma—How Much Fetal Monitoring and Cesarean Section is Enough?" *New England Journal of Medicine* 315(10), 1986.

Gilstrap, L. C., et al. "Cesarean Section: Changing Incidence and Indications." *Obstetrics & Gynecology* 63(2), 1984.

Gleicher, Norman. "Cesarean Section Rates in the United States—The Short-Term Failure of the National Consensus Development Conference in 1980." *Journal of the American Medical Association* 252(23), 1984.

Golde, Steven H. "A Program to Lower Cesarean-Section Rates." *New England Journal of Medicine* 320(25), 1985.

Goldman, Gail, et al. "Factors Influencing the Practice of Vaginal Birth After Cesarean Section." *American Journal of Public Health* 83(8), 1993.

Gould, Jeffrey B., et al. "Socioeconomic Differences in Rates of Cesarean Section." *New England Journal of Medicine* 321(4), 1989.

Goyert, Gregory L., et al. "The Physician Factor in Cesarean Birth Rates." *New England Journal of Medicine* 320(11), 1989.

Greer, A. L. "The State of the Art Versus the State of the Science: The Diffusion of New Medical Technologies into Practice." *International Journal of Technology Assessment in Health Care* 4, 1988.

Haas, Jennifer, et al. "The Effect of Health Coverage for Uninsured Pregnant Women on Maternal Health and the Use of Cesarean Section." *Journal of the American Medical Association* 270(1), 1993.

Haynes de Regt, R., et al. "Relation of Private or Clinic Care to the Cesarean Birth Rate." *New England Journal of Medicine* 315, 1986.

Hornbrook, M. C., and S. E. Berki. "Practice Mode and Payment Method: Effects on Use, Costs, Quality and Access." *Medical Care* 23, 1985.

Hurst, Marsha, and Pamela S. Summey. "Childbirth and Social Class: The Case of Cesarean Delivery." *Social Science and Medicine* 18(8), 1984.

Jeffrey, F., et al. "Maternal Age: An Independent Risk Factor for Cesarean Delivery." *Obstetrics & Gynecology* 81(2), 1993.

Jonas, Harry S. "The Search for a Lower Cesarean Rate Goes On." *Journal of the American Medical Association* 262(11), 1989.

Kizer, Kenneth W., and Art Ellis. "C-Section Rate Related to Payment Source." *American Journal of Public Health* 78(1), 1988.

Kosecoff, Jacqueline, et al. "Effects of the National Institutes of Health Consensus Development Program on Physician Practice." *Journal of the American Medical Association* 258(19), 1987.

Lagrew, D. C., Jr., and M. A. Morgan. "Decreasing the Cesarean Section Rate in a Private Hospital: Success Without Mandated Clinical Changes." *American Journal of Obstetrics and Gynecology* 174(1, part 1), 1996.

Leyland, A. "Socioeconomic and Racial Differences in Obstetric Procedures." *American Journal of Public Health* 83(8), 1993.

Localio, A. Russell, et al. "Relationship Between Malpractice Claims and Cesarean Delivery." *Journal of the American Medical Association* 269(3), 1993.

Lomas, Jonathan, et al. "Do Practice Guidelines Guide Practice? The Effect of a Consensus Statement on the Practice of Physicians." *Journal of the*

American Medical Association 321(19), 1989.

Lomas, Jonathan, et al. "Opinion Leaders vs. Audit and Feedback to Implement Practice Guidelines." *Journal of the American Medical Association* 265(17), 1991.

Lomas, Jonathan, et al. "The Role of Evidence in the Consensus Process." *Journal of the American Medical Association* 259(20), 1988.

Macfarlane, Alison, and G. Chamberlain. "What Is Happening to Cesarean Section Rates?" *Lancet* 342, 1993.

McKenzie, Lisa, and Patricia A. Stephenson. "Variation in Cesarean Section Rates Among Hospitals in Washington State." *American Journal of Public Health* 83(8), 1993.

Myers, Stephen A., and Norman Gleicher. "1988 US Cesarean-Section Rate: Good News or Bad?" *New England Journal of Medicine* 323(3), 1990.

Myers, Stephen A., et al. "A Successful Program to Lower Cesarean-Section Rates." *New England Journal of Medicine* 319, 1988.

Notzon, Francis C. "International Differences in the Use of Obstetric Interventions." *Journal of the American Medical Association* 263(24), 1990.

O'Driscoll, Kevin, et al. "Cesarean Section and Perinatal Outcome: Response from the House of Horne." *American Journal of Obstetrics and Gynecology* 158(3, part 1), 1988.

O'Driscoll, Kevin, and Michael Foley. "Correlation of Decrease in Perinatal Mortality and Increase in Cesarean Section Rates." *Obstetrics & Gynecology* 61(1), 1983.

Phillips, R. N., et al. "Physician Bias in Cesarean Sections." *Journal of the American Medical Association* 248(9), 1982.

Shiono, Patricia, et al. "Reasons for the Rising Cesarean Delivery Rates: 1978–1984." *Obstetrics & Gynecology* 69(5), 1987.

Shiono, Patricia, et al. "Recent Trends in Cesarean Birth and Trial of Labor in the United States." *Journal of the American Medical Association* 257 (1987).

Smith, Sandy. "Gravida with Insurance Is More Likely to Have Cesarean, Longer Stay in Hospital Than Self-Paying Patient." *Ob/Gyn News* 18(11), 1983.

Stafford, Randall S. "Alternative Strategies for Controlling Rising Cesarean Section Rates." *Journal of the American Medical Association* 263(5), 1990.

Stafford, Randall S. "Cesarean Section Use and Source of Payment: An Analysis of California Hospital Discharge Abstracts." *American Journal of Public Health* 80(3), 1990.

Stafford, Randall S. "The Impact of Nonclinical Factors on Repeat Cesarean

Section." *Journal of the American Medical Association* 265(1), 1991.

Stafford, Randall S., et al. "Trends in Cesarean Section Use in California, 1983 to 1990." *American Journal of Obstetrics and Gynecology* 168(4), 1993.

Safety and Effectiveness of Midwifery

(See Chapter 5 bibliographic references.)

Too-Big Babies, Postdate Pregnancies, and Labor Inductions

Adair, C. D., et al. "Labor Induction in Patients with Previous Cesarean Section." *American Journal of Perinatology* 12(6), 1995.

American College of Obstetricians and Gynecologists. "ACOG Practice Patterns: Vaginal Delivery After Previous Cesarean Birth." Number 1, August 1995.

Chauhan, S. P., et al. "Parous Patients' Estimate of Birth Weight in Postterm Pregnancy." *Journal of Perinatology* 15(3), 1995.

Davis, R., et al. "The Role of Previous Birthweight on Risk for Macrosomia in a Subsequent Birth." *Epidemiology* 6(6), 1995.

Gonen, Ofer, et al. "Induction of Labor Versus Expectant Management in Macrosomia: A Randomized Study." *Obstetrics & Gynecology* 89(6), 1997.

Korte, Diana. "The Myth of the Due Date." *Mothering*, Fall 1994.

Lipscomb, K. R., et al. "The Outcome of Macrosomic Infants Weighing at Least 4500 Grams: Los Angeles County & University of Southern California Experience." *Obstetrics & Gynecology* 85(4), 1995.

Menticoglou, S. M., et al. "Must Macrosomic Fetuses Be Delivered by the Caesarean Section? A Review of Outcome for 786 Babies Greater than or Equal to 4,500 Grams." *Australian and New Zealand Journal of Obstetrics and Gynaecology* 32(2), 1992.

Miller, D. A., et al. "Vaginal Birth After Cesarean Section in Twin Gestation." *American Journal of Obstetrics and Gynecology* 175(1), 1996.

Pollack, R. N., et al. "Macrosomia in Postdate Pregnancies: The Accuracy of Routine Ultrasonographic Screening." *American Journal of Obstetrics and Gynecology* 167(1), 1992.

Rouse, Dwight J., et al. "The Effectiveness and Costs of Elective Cesarean Delivery for Fetal Macrosomia Diagnoses by Ultrasound." *Journal of the American Medical Association* 276(18), 1996.

Whitehorse, William. "Estimation of Gestational Age." *Lancet* 341 (1993).

Xenakis, Elly M.-J., et al. "Induction of Labor in the Nineties: Conquering the Unfavorable Cervix." *Obstetrics & Gynecology* 90(2), 1997.

Turning a Breech Baby

Brocks, V., et al. "A Randomized Trial of External Cephalic Version with Tocolysis in Late Pregnancy." *British Journal of Obstetrics and Gynecology* 91 (1984).

Clay, L. S., et al. "External Cephalic Version." *Journal of Nurse-Midwifery* 38(2), 1993.

Gifford, D. S., et al. "Reductions in Cost and Cesarean Rate by Routine Use of External Cephalic Version: A Decision Analysis." *Obstetrics & Gynecology* 85(6), 1995.

Hellstrom, A. C., et al. "When Does External Cephalic Version Succeed?" *Acta Obstetricia et Gynecologica Scandinavica* 69(4), 1990.

Laros, R. K., Jr., et al. "Management of Term Breech Presentation: A Protocol of External Cephalic Version and Selective Trial of Labor." *American Journal of Obstetrics and Gynecology* 172(6), 1995.

Schachter, M., et al. "External Cephalic Version After Previous Cesarean Section—A Clinical Dilemma." *International Journal of Gynaecology and Obstetrics* 45(1), 1994.

Zhang, J., et al. "Efficacy of External Cephalic Version: A Review." *Obstetrics & Gynecology* 82(2), 1993.

Chapter 4. Make the Most of Your Medical Insurance

Anders, George. "Don't Take No... If at First They Turn You Down, Try, Try, Again." *Wall Street Journal,* October 24, 1996.

Awaakye, Barbara. Correspondence with information officer at the American College of Obstetricians and Gynecologists, Washington, DC, March 10, 1997.

Brooks, Andree. "Hiring a Consultant to Do Battle When a Medical Bill Seems Unfair." *New York Times,* November 14, 1996.

"CDC Reports on Childbearing, Reproductive Health." *The Nations' Health,* July 1997.

Freudenheim, Milt. "Some HMOs Find Value in Removing Gatekeepers." *New York Times,* February 2, 1997.

Gardner, Laura B. "Economic Considerations in Cesarean Section Use," in Bruce L. Flamm and Edward J. Quilligan, eds., *Cesarean Section: Guidelines for Appropriate Utilization* (New York: Springer-Verlag, 1995).

Hotelling, Barbara A., and Cheri B. Grant. "Third-Party Reimbursement."

Childbirth Forum, Summer 1995.

Kilborn, Peter T. "Workers Getting Greater Freedom in Health Plans." *New York Times,* August 17, 1997.

Lohse, Deborah. "Prospective Parents Should Look Out for Gaps in Maternity Health Coverage." *Wall Street Journal,* May 3, 1994.

Meckler, Laura. "Study: Most Workers Under Managed Care." *Health Affairs* January 1997.

Thorp, James, and Ginger Breedlove. "Epidural Analgesia in Labor: An Evaluation of Risks and Benefits." *Birth* 23(2), 1995.

"Trends in Length of Stay for Hospital Deliveries—United States, 1970–1992." *Morbidity and Mortality Weekly Review* 4(17), 1995.

Wines, Michael, and Robert Pear. "President Finds Net Advantage from Failure of Health-Care Effort." *New York Times,* July 30, 1995.

Wright, John W., general ed. *The Universal Almanac* (Kansas City, MO: Andrews & McMeel, 1996).

Chapter 5. Find a VBAC-Friendly Doctor or Midwife

Doctors and Midwives

Blanchette, H. "Comparison of Obstetric Outcome of a Primary-Care Access Clinic Staffed by Certified Nurse-Midwives and a Private Practice Group of Obstetricians in the Same Community." *American Journal of Obstetrics and Gynecology* 172(6), 1995.

Buhler, Lynn, et al. "Prenatal Care: A Comparative Evaluation of Nurse-Midwives and Family Physicians." *Canadian Medical Association Journal* 139, 1988.

Butler, J., et al. "Supportive Nurse-Midwife Care Is Associated with a Reduced Incidence of Cesarean Section." *American Journal of Obstetrics and Gynecology* 168(5), 1993.

Davis, L. G., et al. "Cesarean Section Rates in Low-Risk Private Patients Managed by Certified Nurse-Midwives and Obstetricians." *Journal of Nurse-Midwifery* 39(2), 1994.

DeClercq, Eugene R. "Midwifery Care and Medical Complications: The Role of Risk Screening." *Birth* 22(2), 1995.

Fullerton, J. T., et al. "Practice Styles: A Comparison of Obstetricians and Nurse-Midwives." *Journal of Nurse-Midwifery* 41(3), 1996.

Harvey, S., et al. "A Randomized, Controlled Trial of Nurse-Midwifery Care." *Birth* 23(3), 1996.

Hueston, W. J., and M. Rudy. "A Comparison of Labor and Delivery Management Between Nurse Midwives and Family Physicians." *Journal of Family Practice* 37(5), 1993.

Oakley, Deborah, et al. "Processes of Care: Comparisons of Certified Nurse-Midwives and Obstetricians." *Journal of Nurse-Midwifery* 40(5), 1995.

Sakala, C. "Midwifery Care and Out-of-Hospital Birth Settings: How Do They Reduce Unnecessary Cesarean Section Births?" *Social Science and Medicine* 37(10), 1993.

Turan, C., and B. Kutlay. "Cesarean Section Rates and Perinatal Outcomes in Resident and Midwife Attended Low Risk Deliveries." *European Journal of Obstetrics, Gynecology, & Reproductive Biology* 62(1), 1995.

Turnbull, Deborah, et al. "Randomized, Controlled Trial of Efficacy of Midwife-Managed Care." *Lancet* 348, 1996.

If Midwives Are So Great...

Anderson, R., and D. Greener. "A Descriptive Analysis of Home Births Attended by CNMs in Two Nurse-Midwifery Services." *Journal of Nurse-Midwifery* 36(2), 1991.

Bastian, H. "Personal Beliefs and Alternative Childbirth Choices: A Survey of 552 Women Who Planned to Give Birth at Home." *Birth* 20(4), 1993.

Cunningham, J. D. "Experiences of Australian Mothers Who Gave Birth Either at Home, at a Birth Centre, or in Hospital Labour Wards." *Social Science and Medicine* 36(4), 1993.

Malpractice Influences on Whether You Have a VBAC or Another Cesarean

American College of Obstetricians and Gynecologists. "Professional Liability and Its Effects: Report of a 1990 Survey of ACOG's Membership," August 1990.

American College of Obstetricians and Gynecologists. "Vaginal Birth After Cesarean Section: Report of a 1990 Survey of ACOG's Membership," August 1990.

Beckman, H. B., et al. "The Doctor-Patient Relationship and Malpractice: Lessons from Plaintiff Depositions." *Archives of Internal Medicine* 154(12), 1994.

Hickson, Gerald B., et al. "Factors That Prompted Families to File Medical Malpractice Claims Following Perinatal Injuries." *Journal of the American Medical Association* 267(10), 1992.

Levinson, Wendy, et al. "Physician-Patient Communication." *Journal of the American Medical Association* 277(7), 1997.

Localio, A. R., et al. "Relationship Between Malpractice Claims and Cesarean Delivery." *Journal of the American Medical Association* 269(3), 1993.

McCormick, Brian. "Most Doctors Say They Practice Defensive Medicine," *American Medical News,* May 25, 1992.

Obstetricians and Family Physicians

Applegate, J. A., and M. F. Walhout. "Cesarean Section Rate: A Comparison Between Family Physicians and Obstetricians." *Family Practice Research Journal* 12(3), 1992.

Blanchette, H. "Comparison of Obstetric Outcome of a Primary-Care Access Clinic Staffed by Certified Nurse-Midwives and a Private Practice Group of Obstetricians in the Same Community." *American Journal of Obstetrics and Gynecology* 172(6), 1995.

Deutchman, M. E., et al. "Perinatal Outcomes: A Comparison Between Family Physicians and Obstetricians." *Journal of the American Board of Family Practice* 8(6), 1995.

Guillemette, J., and W. D. Fraser. "Differences Between Obstetricians in Caesarean Section Rates and the Management of Labour." *British Journal of Obstetrics and Gynaecology* 99(2), 1992.

Hueston, W. J., et al. "Practice Variations Between Family Physicians and Obstetricians in the Management of Low-Risk Pregnancies." *Journal of Family Practice* 40(4), 1995.

Hueston, W. J., and M. Rudy. "A Comparison of Labor and Delivery Management Between Nurse Midwives and Family Physicians." *Journal of Family Practice* 37(5), 1993.

MacDonald, S. E., et al. "A Comparison of Family Physicians' and Obstetricians' Intrapartum Management of Low-Risk Pregnancies." *Journal of Family Practice* 37(5), 1993.

Out-of-Hospital VBACs and the Risk for Uterine Rupture

Flamm, Bruce L. "Once a Cesarean, Always a Controversy." *Obstetrics & Gynecology* 90, 1997.

Flamm, Bruce L. Personal communication, Riverside, CA, August 1997.

Jones, R. O., et al. "Rupture of Low Transverse Cesarean Scars During Trial of Labor." *Obstetrics & Gynecology* 77, 1991.

Leung, Anna S., et al. "Risk Factors Associated with Uterine Rupture During Trial of Labor After Cesarean Delivery: A Case Control Study." *American*

Journal of Obstetrics and Gynecology 168(6), 1993.

Swan, Farra. Personal communication, Tempe, AZ, May 1995.

Question 1 (for a Doctor): Approximately How Many VBACs Have You Attended?

American College of Obstetricians and Gynecologists. "Vaginal Birth After Cesarean Section: Report of a 1990 Survey of ACOG's Membership," August 28, 1990.

(See "Women Who Want Elective Repeat Cesareans" in Chapter 2 bibliographic references.)

Question 4 (for a Doctor): What Is Your Cesarean Rate?

Burns, L. R., et al. "The Effect of Physician Factors on the Cesarean Section Decision." *Medical Care* 33(4), 1995.

Goldman, G., et al. "Factors Influencing the Practice of Vaginal Birth After Cesarean Section." *American Journal of Public Health* 83(8), 1993.

Tussing, A. D., and M. A. Wojtowycz. "The Effect of Physician Characteristics on Clinical Behavior: Cesarean Section in New York State." *Social Science and Medicine* 37(10), 1993.

Question 5 (for a Doctor): How Do You Usually Manage a Postdate Pregnancy or a Suspected CPD?

Hueston, W. J. "Specialty Differences in Primary Cesarean Section Rates in a Rural Hospital." *Family Practice Research Journal* 12(3), 1992.

Korte, Diana. "The Myth of the Due Date." *Mothering,* Fall 1994.

Question 6 (for a Doctor): What's a Reasonable Length of Time for a VBAC Labor If I'm Healthy and My Baby Appears to Be Healthy?

Paterson, C. M., and N. J. Saunders. "Mode of Delivery After One Caesarean Section: Audit of Current Practice in a Health Region." *British Medical Journal* 303(6806), 1991.

Safety and Effectiveness of Midwifery

Aaronson, L. S. "Nurse-Midwives and Obstetricians: Alternative Models of Care and Client 'Fit'." *Research in Nursing & Health* 10(4), 1987.

Abernathy, Thomas J., and Donna M. Lentjes. "Planned and Unplanned Home Births and Hospital Births in Calgary, Alberta, 1984–87." *Public Health Reports* 104(4), 1989.

Acheson, Louise A., et al. "Patient Selection and Outcomes for Out-of-Hospital Births in One Family Practice." *Journal of Family Practice* 31(2), 1990.

Adamson, G. David, and Douglas J. Gare. "Home or Hospital Births?" *Journal of the American Medical Association* 243(17), 1980.

Anderson, Rondi E., and Patricia Murphy. "Outcomes of 11,788 Planned Home Births Attended by CNMs: A Retrospective Descriptive Study." *Journal of Nurse-Midwifery* 40(6), 1995.

Annandale, Ellen C. "Dimensions of Patient Control in a Free-Standing Birth Center." *Social Science and Medicine* 25(11), 1987.

Baruffi, G., et al. "Investigation of Institutional Differences in Primary Cesarean Birth Rates." *Journal of Nurse-Midwifery* 35(5), 1990.

Beal, M. W. "Nurse-Midwifery Intrapartum Management." *Journal of Nurse-Midwifery* 29(1), 1984.

Blanchette, H. "Comparison of Obstetric Outcome of a Primary-Care Access Clinic Staffed by Certified Nurse-Midwives and a Private Practice Group of Obstetricians in the Same Community." *American Journal of Obstetrics and Gynecology* 172(6), 1995.

Buhler, Lynn, et al. "Prenatal Care: A Comparative Evaluation of Nurse-Midwives and Family Physicians." *Canadian Medical Association Journal* 139, 1988.

Burnett, C. A., et al. "Home Delivery and Neonatal Mortality in North Carolina." *Journal of the American Medical Association* 244(24), 1988.

Butler, J., et al. "Supportive Nurse-Midwife Care Is Associated with a Reduced Incidence of Cesarean Section." *American Journal of Obstetrics and Gynecology* 168(5), 1993.

Butter, Irene H., and B. J. Kay. "State Laws and the Practice of Lay Midwifery." *American Journal of Public Health* 78(9), September 1988.

Campbell, R., and A. MacFarlane. "Place of Delivery: A Review." *British Journal of Obstetrics and Gynaecology* 93(7), 1986.

Cavero, C. M., et al. "Assessment of the Process and Outcomes of the First 1,000 Births of a Nurse-Midwifery Service." *Journal of Nurse-Midwifery* 36(2), 1991.

Chapman, M.G., et al. "The Use of a Birthroom: A Randomised Controlled Trial Comparing Delivery with That in the Labour Ward." *British Journal of Obstetrics and Gynaecology* 93(2), 1986.

Crotty, M., et al. "Planned Homebirths in South Australia 1976–1987." *Medical Journal of Australia* 153, 1990.

Declercq, Eugene R. "The Transformation of American Midwifery: 1975 to

1988." *American Journal of Public Health* 82(5), 1992.

Declercq, Eugene R. "The Trials of Hanna Porn: The Campaign to Abolish Midwifery in Massachusetts." *American Journal of Public Health* 84(6), 1994.

deHaan, J., and F. Smits. "Home Deliveries in the Netherlands: Present Situation and Sequelae." *Journal of Perinatal Medicine* 11, 1983.

Durand, Mark. "The Safety of Home Birth: The Farm Study." *American Journal of Public Health* 82(3), 1992.

Eskes, T. K. "Home Deliveries in the Netherlands—Perinatal Mortality and Morbidity." *International Journal of Gynaecology and Obstetrics* 38(3), 1992.

Feldman, Elizabeth, and M. Hurst. "Outcome and Procedures in Low Risk Birth: A Comparison of Hospital and Birth Center Settings." *Birth* 14(1), 1987.

Ford, Christine, et al. "Outcome of Planned Home Births in an Inner City Practice." *British Medical Journal* 303, 1991.

Fullerton, J. T., and R. Severino. "In-Hospital Care for Low-Risk Childbirth: Comparison with Results from the National Birth Center Study." *Journal of Nurse-Midwifery* 37(5), 1992.

Giles, W., et al. "Antenatal Care of Low Risk Obstetric Patients by Midwives: A Randomised Controlled Trial." *Medical Journal of Australia* 157(3), 1992.

Haire, Doris. "Improving the Outcome of Pregnancy Through Increased Utilization of Midwives." *Journal of Nurse-Midwifery* 6, 1981.

Haire, Doris B., and C. C. Elsberry. "Maternity Care and Outcomes in a High-Risk Service: The North Central Bronx Hospital Experience." *Birth* 18(1), 1991.

Hewitt, M. A., and K. L. Hangsleben. "Nurse-Midwives in a Hospital Birth Center." *Journal of Nurse-Midwifery* 26(5), 1981.

Hinds, M. Ward, et al. "Neonatal Outcome in Planned v. Unplanned Out-of-Hospital Births in Kentucky." *Journal of the American Medical Association* 253(11), 1987.

Hoff, Gerald A. "Having Babies At Home: Is It Safe? Is It Ethical?" *Hastings Center Report* 15(6), 1985.

Howe, K. "Home Births in South-West Australia." *Medical Journal of Australia* 149, 1988.

Hundley, V. A., et al. "Midwife Managed Delivery Unit: A Randomised Controlled Comparison with Consultant Led Care." *British Medical Journal* 309, 1994.

Huygen, F. J. "Home Deliveries in Holland." *Journal of the Royal College of General Practitioners* 34 (1984).

Janssen, Patricia A., et al. "Licensed Midwife Attended, Out of Hospital Births in Washington State: Are They Safe?" *Birth* 21(3), 1994.

Kaufman, K., and H. McDonald. "A Retrospective Evaluation of a Model of Midwifery Care." *Birth* 15(2), 1988.

Kay, Bonnie, et al. "Women's Health and Social Change: The Case of Lay Midwives." *International Journal of Health Services* 18(2), 1988.

Keleher, K. C., and L. Mann. "Nurse-Midwifery Care in an Academic Health Center." *Journal of Obstetric, Gynecologic, and Neonatal Nursing* 15(5), 1986.

Klee, L. "Home Away from Home: The Alternative Birth Center." *Social Science and Medicine* 23(1), 1986.

Klein, M., et al. "A Comparison of Low Risk Pregnant Women Booked for Delivery in Two Systems of Care: Shared Care (Consultant) and Integrated General Practice Unit." *British Journal of Obstetrics and Gynaecology* 90, 1983.

Korte, Diana. "Infant Mortality: Lessons from Japan." *Mothering*, Winter 1992.

Mayes, F., et al. "A Retrospective Comparison of Certified Nurse-Midwife and Physician Management of Low Risk Births: A Pilot Study." *Journal of Nurse-Midwifery* 32(4), 1987.

Mehl, Lewis, et al. "Evaluation of Outcomes of Non–Nurse Midwives: Matched Comparisons with Physicians." *Women & Health* 5, 1980.

Mehl, Lewis, et al. "Outcomes of Elective Home Births: A Series of 1,146 Cases." *Journal of Reproductive Medicine* 19(5), 1977.

Morse, J. M., and C. Park. "Home Birth and Hospital Deliveries: A Comparison of the Perceived Painfulness of Parturition." *Research in Nursing and Health* 11(3), 1988.

Nichols, C. W. "The Yale Nurse Midwifery Practice: Addressing the Outcomes." *Journal of Nurse-Midwifery* 30(3), 1985.

Oppenheimer, Christina. "Organising Midwifery Led Care in the Netherlands." *British Medical Journal* 307, 1993.

Platt, L. D., et al. "Nurse-Midwifery in a Large Teaching Hospital." *Obstetrics & Gynecology* 66(6), 1985.

Reinke, C. "Outcomes of the First 527 Births at the Birthplace in Seattle." *Birth* 9(4), 1982.

Rooks, Judith P., et al. "The National Birth Center Study Part III." *Journal of Nurse-Midwifery* 37 (1992).

Rooks, Judith P., et al. "Outcomes of Care in Birth Centers: The National Birth Center Study." *New England Journal of Medicine* 321(26), 1989.

Rosenblatt, Roger A., et al. "Interspeciality Differences in the Obstetric Care of Low-Risk Women." *American Journal of Public Health* 87(3), 1997.

Sakala, C. "Content of Care by Independent Midwives: Assistance with Pain in Labor and Birth." *Social Science and Medicine* 26(11), 1988.

Sakala, C. "Midwifery Care and Out-of-Hospital Birth Settings: How Do They Reduce Unnecessary Cesarean Section Births?" *Social Science and Medicine* 37(10), 1993.

Schimmel, L. M., et al. "The Yolo County Midwifery Service: A Descriptive Study of 496 Singleton Birth Outcomes, 1990." *Journal of Nurse-Midwifery* 37(6), 1992.

Schramm, W. F., et al. "Neonatal Mortality in Missouri Home Births, 1978–1984." *American Journal of Public Health* 77(8), 1987.

Schreier, A. C. "The Tucson Nurse-Midwifery Service: The First Four Years." *Journal of Nurse-Midwifery* 28(6), 1983.

Scupholme, A., et al. "Nurse-Midwifery Care to Vulnerable Populations. Phase I: Demographic Characteristics of the National CNM Sample." *Journal of Nurse-Midwifery* 37(5), 1992.

Soderstrom, Bobbi, et al. "Interest in Alternative Birthplaces Among Women in Ottawa-Carleton." *Canadian Medical Association Journal* 142(9), 1990.

Stewart, Richard B., and Linda Clark. "Nurse-Midwifery Practice in an In-Hospital Birthing Center: 2050 Births." *Journal of Nurse-Midwifery* 27(3), 1982.

Sullivan, D.A., and R. Beeman. "Four Years' Experience with Home Birth by Licensed Midwives in Arizona." *American Journal of Public Health* 73(6), 1983.

Taylor, Donald H., Jr. "Helping Nurse-Midwives Provide Obstetrical Care in Rural North Carolina." *American Journal of Public Health* 83(6), 1993.

Tew, Marjorie. "Do Obstetric Intranatal Interventions Make Birth Safer?" *British Journal of Obstetrics and Gynaecology* 93, 1986.

Tew, Marjorie. "Place of Birth and Perinatal Mortality." *Journal of the Royal College of General Practitioners*, August 1985.

Tew, Marjorie. "The Practices of Birth Attendants and the Safety of Birth." *Midwifery* 2, 1986.

Tew, Marjorie. *Safer Childbirth? A Critical History of Maternity Care* (London: Chapman and Hall, 1994).

Tew, Marjorie, and S. M. I. Damstra-Wijmenga. "Safest Birth Attendants: Recent Dutch Evidence." *Midwifery* 7, 1991.

Treffers, Pieter E., et al. "Home Births and Minimal Medical Interventions."

224 of THE VBAC COMPANION

Journal of the American Medical Association 264(17), 1990.

Tyson, H. "Outcomes of 1001 Midwife-Attended Home Births in Toronto, 1983–1988." *Birth* 18(1), 1991.

van Alten, D., et al. "Midwifery in the Netherlands, the Wormerveer Study: Selection, Mode of Delivery, Perinatal Mortality and Infant Morbidity. *British Journal of Obstetrics and Gynaecology* 96(6), 1989.

Two Kinds of U.S. Midwives

Korte, Diana. "Midwives on Trial." *Mothering,* Fall 1995.

Notzon, Francis C., et al. "International Differences in the Use of Obstetric Interventions." *Journal of the American Medical Association* 263(24), 1990.

Patamia, Kimberly. Interview with information director, American College of Nurse-Midwives, January 28, 1997.

Chapter 6. Find a VBAC-Friendly Hospital or Birth Center

Birth Centers

Harrington, L. C., et al. "Vaginal Birth After Cesarean in a Hospital-Based Birth Center Staffed by Certified Nurse-Midwives." *Journal of Nurse-Midwifery* 42(4), 1997.

Rooks, Judith P., et al. "Outcomes of Care in Birth Centers: The National Birth Center Study." *New England Journal of Medicine* 321(26), 1989.

Shaw, I. "Reaction to Transfer Out of a Hospital Birth Center: A Pilot Study." *Birth* 12(3), 1985.

Electronic Fetal Monitor

Elkin, Murray, et al. *A Guide to Effective Care in Pregnancy and Childbirth.* (Oxford, England: Oxford University Press, 1995).

Flamm, Bruce L. "Electronic Fetal Monitoring in the United States." *Birth* 21(2) 1994.

Freeman, Roger. "Intrapartum Fetal Monitoring—A Disappointing Story." *New England Journal of Medicine* 322(9), 1990.

Neilson, James P. "Electronic Fetal Heart Rate Monitoring During Labor: Information from Randomized Trials." *Birth* 21(2), 1994.

Placek, Paul J. "Electronic Fetal Monitoring in Relation to Cesarean Section Delivery, for Live Births and Stillbirths in the U.S., 1980." *Public Health Reports* 99(2), 1984.

Following are the nine randomized controlled trials that are the basis for the statement that EFM has failed to benefit either babies or mothers:

1. Haverkamp, A. D., et al. "The Evaluation of Continuous Fetal Heart Rate Monitoring in High-Risk Pregnancy." *American Journal of Obstetrics and Gynecology* 125, 1976.

2. Renou, P., et al. "Controlled Trial of Fetal Intensive Care." *American Journal of Obstetrics and Gynecology* 126, 1976.

3. Kelso, I. M., et al. "An Assessment of Continuous Fetal Heart Rate Monitoring in Labor: A Randomized Trial." *American Journal of Obstetrics and Gynecology* 131, 1978.

4. Haverkamp, A. D., et al. "A Controlled Trial of the Differential Effects of Intrapartum Fetal Monitoring." *American Journal of Obstetrics and Gynecology* 134, 1981.

5. Wood, C., et al. "A Controlled Trial of Fetal Heart Rate Monitoring in a Low-Risk Obstetric Population." *American Journal of Obstetrics and Gynecology* 1134, 1981.

6. MacDonald, D., et al. "The Dublin Randomized Controlled Trial of Intrapartum Fetal Heart Rate Monitoring." *American Journal of Obstetrics and Gynecology* 152, 1985.

7. Leveno, K. J., et al. "A Prospective Comparison of Selective and Universal Electronic Fetal Monitoring in 34,995 Pregnancies." *New England Journal of Medicine* 315(10), 1986.

8. Luthy, D. A., et al. "A Randomized Trial of Electronic Fetal Monitoring in Preterm Labor." *Obstetrics & Gynecology* 69(5), 1987.

9. Shy, K. K., et al. "Effects of Electronic Fetal-Heart-Rate Monitoring, as Compared with Periodic Auscultation, on the Neurologic Development of Premature Infants." *New England Journal of Medicine* 322(9), 1990.

Question 1: What Is the VBAC Rate at Your Hospital?

Coulder, Christopher H., and Richard Lehrfeld. "When Push Comes to Shove: Implementing VBAC Practice Guidelines." *Physician Executive,* June 1995.

Oleske, D. M., et al. "The Cesarean Birth Rate: Influence of Hospital Teaching Status." *Health Services Research* 26(3), 1991.

Pennsylvania Health Care Cost Containment Council. "Northcentral Pennsylvania C-Section and VBAC Information by Hospital." From the Internet, July 1996.

Question 4: What Is the Cesarean Rate at Your Hospital?

Gordon, G. S., et al. "Charges for Comprehensive Obstetric Care at Teaching and Nonteaching Hospitals: A Comparison." *Western Journal of Medicine* 155(6), 1991.

McKenzie, L., and P. A. Stephenson. "Variation in Cesarean Section Rates Among Hospitals in Washington State." *American Journal of Public Health* 83(8), 1993.

Rock, Steven M. "Variability and Consistency of Rates of Primary and Repeat Cesarean Sections Among Hospitals in Two States." *Public Health Reports* 108(4), 1993.

Question 5: What Is the Nurse-Patient Ratio at Your Hospital?

Awaakye, Barbara. Correspondence with information officer at the American College of Obstetricians and Gynecologists, Washington, DC, February and March 1997.

Radin, T. G., et al. "Nurses' Care During Labor: Its Effect on the Cesarean Birth Rate of Healthy, Nulliparous Women." *Birth* 20(1), 1993.

Swirsky, Joan. "Hospitals Downsize R.N.–Patient Ratio." *Wall Street Journal*, April 5, 1996.

Chapter 7. Work with Your Other VBAC Helpers

Doulas and Birth Assistants

Hodnett, Ellen D., and Richard W. Osborn. "A Randomized Trial of the Effects of Monitrice Support During Labor: Mothers' Views Two to Four Weeks Postpartum." *Birth* 16(4), 1989.

Kennel, John H., et al. "Continuous Emotional Support During Labor. A Randomized Controlled Trial." *Journal of the American Medical Association* 265(17), 1991.

Klaus, Marshall, et al. "Effects of Social Support During Parturition on Maternal and Infant Morbidity." *British Medical Journal* 293, 1986.

Sosa, Roberto, et al. "The Effect of a Supportive Woman on Mothering Behavior and the Duration and Complications of Labor." *Pediatric Research* 13, 1979.

Chapter 8. Experience a VBAC Labor

Breaking the Bag of Waters—Amniotomy

Brisson-Carroll, G., et al. "The Effect of Routine Early Amniotomy on

Spontaneous Labor: A Meta-Analysis." *Obstetrics & Gynecology* 87 (5, part 2), 1996.

Enemas

Romney, M. L., and H. Gordon. "Is Your Enema Really Necessary?" *British Medical Journal* 282, 1981.

Epidurals and Cesareans

Haire, Doris. "Obstetric Drugs: Their Effects on Mother and Infant." Alliance for the Improvement of Maternity Services (http://www.comet.net/aims/rothdrug.html), 1997.

Kaminski, H. M., et al. "The Effect of Epidural Analgesia on the Frequency of Instrumental Obstetric Delivery." *Obstetrics & Gynecology* 69(5), 1987.

Lieberman, E., et al. "Epidural Analgesia, Intrapartum Fever, and Neonatal Sepsis Evaluation." *Pediatrics* 99(3), 1997.

MacArthur, C., et al. "Epidural Anaesthesia and Long-Term Backache After Childbirth." *British Medical Journal* 301, 1990.

MacArthur, C., et al. "Investigation of Long Term Problems After Obstetric Epidural Anaesthesia." *British Medical Journal* 304, 1992.

Marttila, M., et al. "Maternal Half-Sitting Position in the Second Stage of Delivery." *Obstetrics & Gynecology* 69(5), 1987.

Thorp, James A., et al. "The Effect of Intrapartum Epidural Anesthesia on Nulliparous Labor: A Randomized Controlled, Prospective Trial." *American Journal of Obstetrics and Gynecology* 169(4), 1993.

Thorp, James A., et al. "Epidural Analgesia in Labor and Cesarean Delivery for Dystocia." *Obstetrical and Gynecological Survey* 49(5), 1994.

Thorp, James A., et al. "Epidural Anesthesia and Cesarean Section for Dystocia: Risk Factors in Nulliparas." *American Journal of Perinatology* 8(6), 1991.

Thorp, James A., and Ginger Breedlove. "Epidural Analgesia in Labor: An Evaluation of Risks and Benefits." *Birth* 23(2), 1996.

Morton, S. C., et al. "Effect of Epidural Analgesia for Labor on the Cesarean Delivery Rate." *Obstetrics & Gynecology* 83(6), 1994.

Episiotomy

Banta, H. David, and Stephen B. Thacker. "The Case for Reassessment of Health Care Technology." *Journal of the American Medical Association* 264(2), 1990.

Henricksen, Tine B., et al. "Methods and Consequences of Changes in Use of Episiotomy." *British Medical Journal* 309, 1994.

Klein, Michael, et al. "Relationship of Episiotomy to Perineal Trauma and Morbidity, Sexual Dysfunction, and Pelvic Floor Relaxation." *American Journal of Obstetrics and Gynecology* 171(3), 1994.

Sultan, A. H., et al. "Third Degree Obstetric Anal Sphincter Tears: Risk Factors and Outcome of Primary Repair." *British Medical Journal* 308, 1994.

Pain-Relieving Techniques for Labor

Carbonne, B., et al. "Maternal Position During Labor: Effects on Fetal Oxygen Saturation Measured by Pulse Oximetry." *Obstetrics & Gynecology* 88(5), 1996.

Golay, J., et al. "The Squatting Position for the Second Stage of Labor: Effects on Labor and on Maternal and Fetal Well-Being." *Birth* 20(2), 1993.

Lieberman, Adrienne B. *Easing Labor Pain* (Boston: Harvard Common Press, 1992).

Korte, Diana. *Every Woman's Body* (New York: Ballantine Books, 1994).

Sammons, Lucy N. "The Use of Music by Women During Childbirth." *Journal of Nurse-Midwifery* 29(4), 1984.

Perineal Massage

Labrecque, Michel, et al. "Prevention of Perineal Trauma by Perineal Massage During Pregnancy: A Pilot Study." *Birth* 21(1), 1994.

Mynaugh, P. A. "A Randomized Study of Two Methods of Teaching Perineal Massage: Effects on Practice Rates, Episiotomy Rates, and Lacerations." *Birth* 18(3), 1991.

Phases of Labor

Albers, Leah, et al. "The Length of Active Labor in Normal Pregnancies." *Obstetrics & Gynecology* 87(3), 1996.

Friedman, Emmanuel A. "The Graphic Analysis of Labor." *American Journal of Obstetrics and Gynecology* 68, 87(3), 1954.

Gemer, O., et al. "Detection of Scar Dehiscence at Delivery in Women with Prior Cesarean Section." *Acta Obstetricia et Gynecologica Scandinavica* 71(7), 1992.

Harlass, F. E., and P. Duff. "The Duration of Labor in Primiparas Undergoing Vaginal Birth After Cesarean Delivery." *Obstetrics & Gynecology* 75(1), 1990.

Kaplan, B., et al. "Routine Revision of Uterine Scar After Prior Cesarean Section." *Acta Obstetricia et Gynecologica Scandinavica* 73(6), 1994.

Korte, Diana. *Every Woman's Body* (New York: Ballantine Books, 1994).

Korte, Diana, and Roberta Scaer. *A Good Birth, A Safe Birth* (Boston: Harvard Common Press, 1992).

Seitchik, J., et al. "Amniotomy and Oxytocin Treatment of Functional Dystocia and Route of Delivery." *American Journal of Obstetrics and Gynecology* 155(3), 1986.

Pitocin or Prostaglandin Gel

Adair, C. D., et al. "Labor Induction in Patients with Previous Cesarean Section." *American Journal of Perinatology* 12(6), 1995.

Blanco, J. D., et al. "Prostaglandin E2 Gel Induction of Patients with a Prior Low Transverse Cesarean Section." *American Journal of Perinatology* 9(2), 1992.

Chelmow, D., and R. K. Laros, Jr. "Maternal and Neonatal Outcomes After Oxytocin Augmentation in Patients Undergoing a Trial of Labor After Prior Cesarean Delivery." *Obstetrics & Gynecology* 80(6), 1992.

Norman, M., and G. Ekman. "Preinductive Cervical Ripening with Prostaglandin E2 in Women with One Previous Cesarean Section." *Acta Obstetricia et Gynecologica Scandinavica* 71(5), 1992.

Sakala, E. P., et al. "Oxytocin Use After Previous Cesarean: Why a Higher Rate of Failed Labor Trial?" *Obstetrics & Gynecology* 75(3, part 1), 1990.

Summers, Lisa. "Methods of Cervical Ripening and Labor Induction." *Journal of Nurse-Midwifery* 42(2), 1997.

Chapter 9. Appreciate Your Birth Experience

Advantages of Surgery with Full-Term Baby After Labor Has Started

(See Chapter 1 bibliographic references for "Birth Canal Hormones," "Born on Time," and "Healthy Lungs.")

Blood Transfusions

Cousins, L. M., et al. "Pre-Cesarean Blood Bank Orders: A Safe and Less Expensive Approach." *Obstetrics & Gynecology* 87(6), 1996.

Cumming, Paul D., et al. "Exposure of Patients to Human Immunodeficiency Virus Through the Transfusion of Blood Components That Test Antibody-Negative." *New England Journal of Medicine* 321(14), 1989.

"Elective Surgery Has Too Many Transfusions, ACP Says." *American Medical News,* March 16, 1992.

Goldsmith, Marsha F. "As More Surgeons Opt for Autologous Transfusion

Route, What's Ahead?" *Journal of the American Medical Association* 262(22), 1989.

Herbert, W. N., et al. "Autologous Blood Storage in Obstetrics." *Obstetrics and Gynecology* 72(2), 1988.

McCullough, Jeffrey. "The Nation's Changing Blood Supply System." *Journal of the American Medical Association* 269(17), 1993.

Naef, R. W., III, et al. "Hemorrhage Associated with Cesarean Delivery: When Is Transfusion Needed?" *Journal of Perinatology* 15(1), 1995.

Salem-Schatz, S. R., et al. "Influence of Clinical Knowledge, Organizational Context, and Practice Style on Transfusion Decision Making: Implications for Practice Change Strategies." *Journal of the American Medical Association* 264(4), 1990.

Silberstein, Leslie, et al. "Strategies for the Review of Transfusion Practices." *Journal of the American Medical Association* 262(14), 1989.

Sloand, Elaine M., et al. "Safety of the Blood Supply." *Journal of the American Medical Association* 274(17), 1995.

"Study Suggests Popularity of Autologous Donation." *American Medical News,* September 14, 1992.

Lower Risk of Infection When Doctor Has Lots of Cesarean Experience

(See Chapter 1 bibliographic references for "Lower Risk for Infection.")

Postpartum Pain Relief

Ho, C. M., et al. "Effect of P-6 Acupressure on Prevention of Nausea and Vomiting After Epidural Morphine for Post-Cesarean Section Pain Relief." *Acta Anaesthesiolica Scandinavica* 40(3), 1996.

Kuhn, S., et al. "Perceptions of Pain Relief After Surgery." *British Medical Journal* 300, 1990.

Lieberman, Adrienne B. *Easing Labor Pain.* (Boston: Harvard Common Press, 1992).

Olden, A. J., et al. "Patients' Versus Nurses' Assessments of Pain and Sedation After Cesarean Section." *Journal of Obstetric, Gynecologic, and Neonatal Nursing* 24(2), 1995.

Surgery Usually Not on Weekends

Clarke, Sally, and Selma Taffel. "Changes in Cesarean Delivery in the United States, 1988 and 1993." *Birth,* June 1995.

Reader Questionnaire

Dear Reader:

Here's a way you can let me know what you think about this book and make suggestions for future editions. Please answer the following questions on separate paper and send them to me, Diana Korte, c/o Harvard Common Press, 535 Albany Street, Boston, MA 02118 or e-mail me at: DianaKorte@aol.com.

1. Why did you have a cesarean?

2. How many cesareans did you have?

3. Did you have a doctor or midwife (CNM or direct entry) for your VBAC?

4. Was your VBAC at a hospital, birth center, or home?

5. Did you have a labor assistant or doula?

6. If you had any worries about having a VBAC, what were they?

7. What individual or resource was most helpful in having a VBAC?

8. What information in this book helped you the most?

9. What was your biggest surprise when you had your VBAC?

10. Is there anything else you'd like to tell me? (Birth stories are welcome.)

Index